A Practical Guide to Fascial Manipulation

For Elsevier

Senior Content Strategist: Rita Demetriou-Swanwick
Content Development Specialist: Nicola Lally
Project Manager: Julie Taylor
Designer/Design Direction: Christian Bilbow
Illustration Manager: Karen Giacomucci
Illustrator: Richard Tibbitts at Antbits

A Practical Guide to Fascial Manipulation

An Evidence- and Clinical-Based Approach

TUULIA LUOMALA PT

Physiotherapist, Lecturer, Teacher, Veterinary Fascial Manipulation Teacher, MT-Physio Oy, Lempäälä, Finland

MIKA PIHLMAN PT

Physiotherapist, Lecturer, Teacher, MT-Physio OY, Lempäälä, Finland

Consulting Technical Editor

CARLA STECCO MD

Orthopaedic Surgeon; Assistant Professor of Human Anatomy and Movement Science, University of Padua, Italy

English Language Editor

WARREN HAMMER DC MS

Postgraduate Faculty, New York Chiropractic College, NY, USA; Northwestern Health Sciences University, Bloomington, MN, USA

Forewords by

LUIGI STECCO PT and CARLA STECCO MD

ELSEVIER

ELSEVIER

ISBN 978-0-7020-6659-7

Notices

Knowledge and best practice in this field are constantly changing. As new research and experience broaden our understanding, changes in research methods, professional practices, or medical treatment may become necessary.

Practitioners and researchers must always rely on their own experience and knowledge in evaluating and using any information, methods, compounds, or experiments described herein. In using such information or methods they should be mindful of their own safety and the safety of others, including parties for whom they have a professional responsibility.

With respect to any drug or pharmaceutical products identified, readers are advised to check the most current information provided (i) on procedures featured or (ii) by the manufacturer of each product to be administered, to verify the recommended dose or formula, the method and duration of administration, and contraindications. It is the responsibility of practitioners, relying on their own experience and knowledge of their patients, to make diagnoses, to determine dosages and the best treatment for each individual patient, and to take all appropriate safety precautions.

To the fullest extent of the law, neither the Publisher nor the authors, contributors, or editors, assume any liability for any injury and/or damage to persons or property as a matter of products liability, negligence or otherwise, or from any use or operation of any methods, products, instructions, or ideas contained in the material herein.

Printed in Great Britain
Last digit is the print number: 10 9 8 7 6 5 4 3

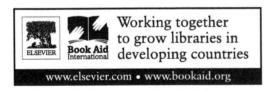

CONTENTS

Companion Website: www.guidefascial.com

- video bank
- image bank

VIDEO LIST

All videos are available on:

www.guidefascial.com

and are identified in the book through the video icon ▶ located on the right of the page and its number in the text.

CHAPTER 1: HISTORY OF FASCIAL MANIPULATION

CHAPTER 2: ANATOMY OF THE FASCIA FROM THE CLINICAL POINT OF VIEW

CHAPTER 3: PHYSIOLOGY OF THE FASCIA FROM THE CLINICAL POINT OF VIEW

CHAPTER 4: FASCIAL MANIPULATION

When Tuulia Luomala told me that she was collaborating with Mika Pihlman to write a book on Fascial Manipulation, I was happy to encourage her. The book was to explain Fascial Manipulation (FM) to healthcare professionals as well as to the general public. As I was aware of Tuulia's commitment, passion, and years of preparation in the study of the fascia, I was convinced that the work would be a significant addition to the field as it would broaden the understanding of recent discoveries in this relatively new field of study.

For decades, even centuries, anatomy and physiology texts have acknowledged the presence of fascia in the body with a few sentences describing its function both as binding anatomical structures together and filling the interstices between them. Recent work has demonstrated that the fascial system plays a far more important role in the biomechanical function of the body than was previously imagined. For instance, we now know that the brain controls movement by commanding changes in all three planes in space, rather than by controlling the function of each individual muscle. The cerebral impulses are organized in a detailed way to a specific muscle in the peripheral fascia.

Terminology has proved a challenge for those studying the fascia as an anatomical system. Depending on its composition, fascia is referred to as latae or aponeurosis. Other fasciae are called by the name of the specific muscle covered (for example, the pectoral fascia) or by the name of the segment in which it is found, like the crural, plantar, brachial, or lumbar fascia. Or, again, by the depth in the body—superficial, medial, and profundus. Some fascia are named for the researcher who first described it (the fascia of Scarpa, Colles, or Buck). None of these names refer to the role fasciae play within the physiology of the musculoskeletal system. This is the reason why it has been necessary to find more specific terms that can logically connect the fascia to movement. In the beginning of this book the reader might find it difficult to use these new terms. However, further study in the field will reveal that these terms agree with the most recent research in neurophysiology. This new terminology will thus facilitate the study of the newest advances and the understanding of the latest treatment modalities of the fascia, such as FM.

This book first presents the fasciae from a microscopic point of view followed by analysis in their macroscopic conformation. The authors explain that some pathological changes in fascial tissue (densification) may exist in the fascial biochemistry but are not observed in the joint tissue itself. This explains why directly treating the joints might not alleviate joint pain. In many cases, looking for the cause of pain in the fascia can suggest more effective treatment strategies. Joint pain is now considered more often a consequence of fascial dysfunction than joint dysfunction. In the early pages of Chapter 4, the text gives guidelines for the healthcare professional to use to trace painful dysfunction to the true source of the pain.

Leonardo da Vinci said that there can be no science without experience. Both authors of this text have absorbed knowledge of the fascia based on their own numerous dissections on human and animal cadavers. Tuulia has applied the treatment of fascial dysfunction in her work on horses and dogs and has extended the value of FM to the veterinary field. She is the first teacher of Veterinary Fascial Manipulation (VFM). For her insight and dedication, I gladly write these lines, confident that Tuulia's and Mika's research will improve and enrich my own endeavours in the field of fascial research and treatment.

I thank both authors for their efforts in introducing FM and making it understandable to an even wider audience. One of the rewards for writing a book is the knowledge that one acquires in its preparation. An even greater reward is the realization that one has helped to alleviate human and animal suffering. The latter was surely the motivating inspiration for this book. And now, dear reader, you have the opportunity to cooperate in this effort by transmitting this knowledge to others. Your grateful patients will be your reward in this noble effort.

Sincerely,
Luigi Stecco, PT

I have known Tuulia and Mika for many years, and I quickly noticed their capacity to communicate and their curiosity about all the fasciae news. They have always demonstrated a great interest in Fascial Manipulation and perseverance in their personal research. For this reason I strongly supported their project to present, in an easy way, the main concepts of the Fascial Manipulation technique. They understood that we still lack a book to introduce the main concepts of Fascial Manipulation to a wider audience. All the published books about Fascial Manipulation were written to explain in detail the technique, but in this way they are limited to a selective audience. Really, many patients, doctors, physiotherapists, osteopaths, manual therapists and movement trainers just want to have some knowledge about Fascial Manipulation and its biomechanical model. This book fills such a gap. Tuulia and Mika were able to transform the 'hard-to-understand' into the 'easy-to-use' to enable learners at every level to fuel their pursuit of professional and personal advancement. This book is an extremely user-friendly book for all those people who are interested to know the main concepts of Fascial Manipulation. The book is clear, concise, readable, it is written in very understandable language with wonderful pictures and anecdotes from the authors. The material is presented in short, easy-to-digest bites. This book is logically organized, beginning with a short history of Fascial Manipulation, then describing the fascial anatomy (Chapter 2) and physiology (Chapter 3). The other chapters are more focused on Fascial Manipulation technique (FM), in particular Chapter 4 presents the key concepts of the FM, Chapter 5 some examples of treatments, Chapter 6 the FM for internal dysfunction and Chapter 8 the FM for veterinary. In this way all the main aspects of FM are presented. Besides, thanks to the revision of Warren Hammer, the book is also easy to read, fluid and clear. Tuulia and Mika have done a great job reviewing basic physiology of fasciae in its relationship to movement, myofascial pain and treatment. This book does not delve too deeply into any topic but gives enough information on many topics that if you want to know more about one you can begin your own research. It is not a technical manual of Fascial Manipulation and used alone cannot define a good treatment for a true patient, but for those of us who are not studying to become a Fascial Manipulation practitioner, this is a very informative book. If you get the chance to go to one of Fascial Manipulation official courses, it could be useful to read this book before being introduced to the argument and to be better able to follow the course. I hope this handbook will be useful to spread to a wider audience the ideas of my father Luigi Stecco. It is 30 years since the publication of Luigi Stecco's first book in Italian, and I am very proud that his ideas have inspired others and also now the books of other authors.

Carla Stecco

ACKNOWLEDGEMENTS

The process of writing this book has involved a network of support and contributions not unlike the fascial network. Many have helped in this great project. International experts were particularly important. Specifically, we could not have done it without the help of Carla Stecco MD PhD and Warren Hammer DC MS. They have been most generous with their time and knowledge. The staff at Elsevier have supported our efforts generously and competently. We would like to single out Rita Demetriou-Swanwick, Nicola Lally and Julie Taylor, without whose efforts this book would never have been ready as a resource for you, the reader, so that you may understand the advances in the exciting new field of Fascial Manipulation. Enjoy!

We are profoundly grateful to Luigi Stecco. Our admiration for this pioneer in the understanding and treatment of the fascial system—Fascial Manipulation—knows no bounds. His enthusiasm for the work and his joy in its on-going development can be seen in the sparkle in his eyes. His clinical experience and scientific research have laid the foundation for and developed this very new treatment approach. Using his diagnosis and treatment methods, patients suffering from a surprising variety of lesions can be helped. Thanks to Fascial Manipulation, many patients can be successfully delivered from pain and helped into lasting wellbeing. Luigi Stecco has given our patients this gift through us and we are honoured to be a part of the process.

Finally, I would like to thank my mom for all of the support that she provided for this project. I hug my son, who has been patient through this lengthy and time-consuming process. And finally, thank you Anna Nurmio for your help and support.

Tuulia

For me, the writing of this book is part of a lifelong process of learning. I am thankful to the many who have helped us along. I want to dedicate this book to everyone willing to learn and understand the human myofascial system more precisely.

Mika

In the end we can say:

Where the spirit does not work with the hand, there is no art

Leonardo da Vinci

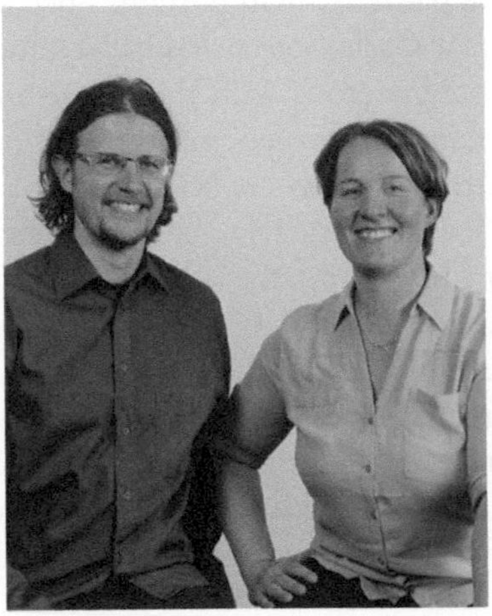

Mika and Tuulia

INTRODUCTION

Luigi Stecco has been developing Fascial Manipulation (FM), the Stecco method, for over 40 years. The method results from years of clinical experience backed by strong scientific research. Over the years both fascial research and clinical studies have validated the importance of this long-overlooked tissue, the fascia. Anatomical, histological, and cadaver studies supported by clinical research have established Fascial Manipulation. It is taught all over the world and many certified instructors are travelling from country to country to educate practitioners.

This book introduces FM in an understandable way to both the practitioner and lay audience. Our journey begins with the history of Fascial Manipulation, followed by the anatomy and physiology of fasciae. Finally we will immerse ourselves into FM and its principles. Fascial Manipulation begins with the patient's interview and it ends with FM treatment. The whole protocol is revealed to help the reader understand the path of the patient in FM. Case examples are provided to expose the ideas behind the clinical reasoning. This book can be used as a teaching guide in FM courses and different conferences. It can be recommended to students and practitioners who have attended Fascial Manipulation courses or it can be useful to those who are thinking of learning FM. This practical guide will provide basic knowledge and understanding about Fascial Manipulation. Hopefully it will inspire people to learn more and increase their understanding of the fascial tensional network and its connections to the cause of many musculoskeletal and internal dysfunctions. In the end, it is hoped to enhance the skill of the practitioner. As Luigi Stecco often says, "*Manus sapiens potens est*": a knowledgeable hand is a more powerful hand.

This is the story of Fascial Manipulation. How do we use it and when do we use it? What are its benefits? When a body is working harmoniously its orchestra will play the most beautiful concerto. If one or more of the instruments are not tuned, the whole orchestra will sound discordant. Our task is to maintain homeostasis of the body. Fascial Manipulation can be the healing tuner of the body.

Welcome to the world of Fascial Manipulation!

Our guide in this book will be Fama. The name Fama comes from the abbreviation of Fascial Manipulation. The word Fama also means in Latin "story" and "report". Fama will pop up in boxes throughout the book showing important thoughts and clinical tips.

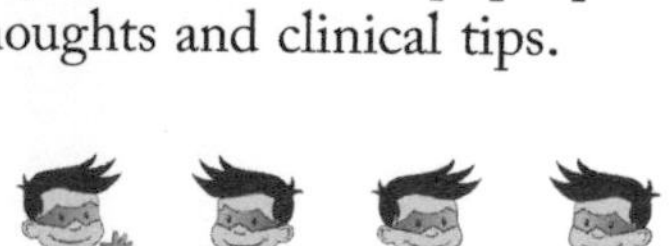

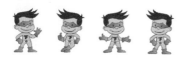

CHAPTER 1

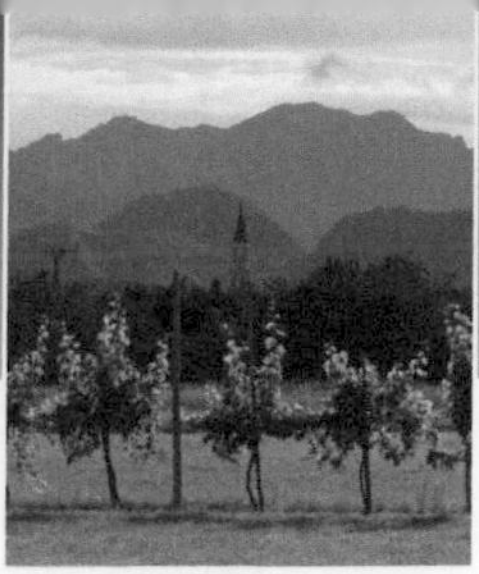

History of Fascial Manipulation

"The most important thing is to be enthusiastic and to have the passion for the work you do."
Luigi Stecco

Italian physiotherapist Luigi Stecco (born in 1949) is the inventor of fascial manipulation (FM). Nothing illustrates his motto better than the image of Luigi Stecco as a boy developing an early fascination for vertebrate anatomy as he dissected a fish his mother had brought home for dinner. Over the next decades, this interest became focused on the thus far little studied but ubiquitous tissue: the fascia. Eventually, the understanding of the fascia as a system—a system with specific vital functions—led Stecco and his colleagues to develop a method of evaluating and treating dysfunctional fascia.

Luigi Stecco has devoted his career to developing and teaching others to develop "knowing hands" in their treatment of pain and dysfunctions. *Manus sapiens, potens est* (a knowledgeable hand is a powerful one). Knowing more will enhance your skills more. Better results in treatments will come with practice and knowledge. In this way FM can be your map of understanding (Fig. 1.1) (see Video 1).

The evolution of FM began over 40 years ago when Luigi was working as a trainee in a hospital. He started developing his own biomechanical model because he realized that many of the treatment techniques he had been taught as a physical therapist were not effective enough—some were even useless. He wanted to find a better way. He started to observe the work bonesetters were doing and realized that they were helping people. However, he was dissatisfied with even these techniques, so he decided to explore different treatments more thoroughly. Luigi gradually started to create his own technique, the Stecco method, later known as FM.

From 1972 to 1984, Luigi worked on his own treatment techniques, building on the inspiration of other treatment methods and basing everything on careful and incessant dissection to gain a profound understanding of anatomical function. He explored osteopathic techniques, then relaxation techniques with the idea that pain could come from psychosomatic factors. Subsequently, he investigated psychomotricity, postural gymnastics, and the Vayer method, which concentrate on dynamic balance and coordination. He was still dissatisfied with the level of clinical results: they were not good enough. He wanted more. He wanted to find a way to turn practitioners' hands into more effective healing hands (Fig. 1.2).

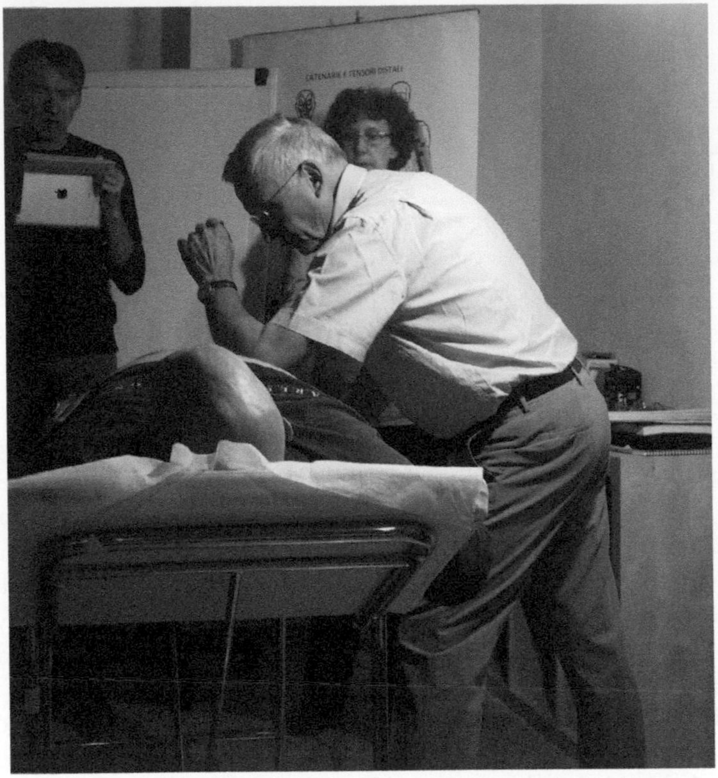

Fig. 1.1 Luigi treating one of the participants in the fascial manipulation course.

In 1976 Luigi was introduced to connective tissue massage and he identifies this as the turning point for meaningful improvement in patient results. This heightened his determination to explore the architecture of connective tissue. He studied the works of Elisabeth Dicke, who was a physiotherapist in Germany in the late 1920s. She especially influenced Luigi's focus on the importance of connective tissue. He became an expert in transverse friction massage. A study of James Cyriax, the father of orthopedic medicine, underscored the importance of the use of the therapist's hands and manual therapy. Combining the knowledge of transverse friction massage and acupuncture meridians confirmed Luigi's theories on the tensional network of the body. The vectorial forces, which act along this network, can be understood and thus lead the practitioner to the areas in the network that need treatment.

Luigi's understanding of the "tensional network" of the human body was enriched by the studies of Ida Rolf and by works on trigger points as elucidated by Travell and Simmons in the early 1980s. The powerful work on kinetic chains

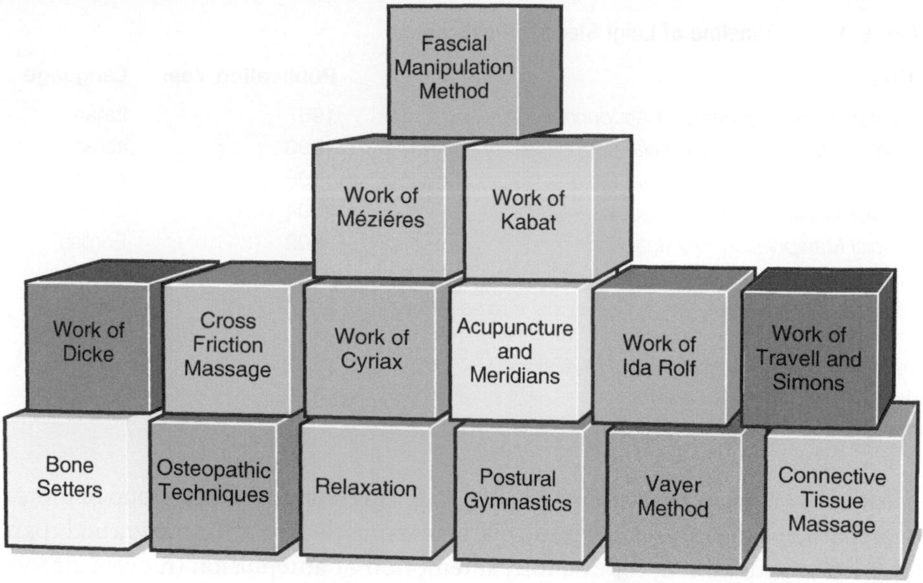

Fig. 1.2 Building blocks of fascial manipulation.

by Francoise Mézières and Herman Kabat was also important in the foundation of Luigi's theoretical understanding. The previous findings and good results from treatments encouraged him to write down all that he had learned through years of clinical experience and studies.

His understanding of the tensional network of the human body had produced good results in clinical settings so Luigi was finally ready to share his insights in his first book, *Myofascial Sequences and Acupuncture Meridians* (1987). At the time, Luigi theorized that the excellent clinical results he was getting were a result of freeing the nerve within the connective tissue, so he named this the "neuroconnective technique." This early technique was the first step in the development of FM as it is known and taught today (Table 1.1).

Luigi continued to study and explore. The anatomic work of Chiarugi, Testut, Gray, and Beninghoff inspired Luigi to deepen his understanding of anatomy. Then, in 1989, at the First International Symposium on Myofascial Pain and Fibromyalgia, the idea of the myofascial unit was launched. At this conference, he presented that points formed the centers of vectors caused by muscular tractions operating within a particular plane of fascia. He wrote that the referral of pain due to these points was related to planes of altered fascia. In the symposium Luigi stated: "Knowing the location of the myofascial unit, it is easier to find the starting point of myofascial pain." This reasoning resulted in what is now defined as the myofascial unit (MFU).

TABLE 1.1 ■ **Timeline of Luigi Stecco's Publications**

Title	Publication Year	Language
Myofascial Sequences and Acupuncture Meridians	1987	Italian
Pain and the Neuromyofascial Sequences	1990	Italian
La Manipolizione Neuroconnectivale	1996	Italian
Fascial Manipulation for Musculoskeletal Pain	2004	English
Fascial Manipulation Practical Part	2009	English
Fascial Manipulation for Internal Dysfunction	2013	English
Manipolazione fasciale per le Disfunzioni Interne—Parte Pratica	2014	Italian
Atlante di Fisiologia della Fascia Muscolare	2016	Italian

An MFU is a key element in FM (Fig. 1.3). It is composed of a group of motor units that activate monoarticular and biarticular muscle fibers that move a body part in a particular direction, for example, antemotion or antepulsion (movement forward in the sagittal direction). The MFU is also composed of nerves (efferent, receptors, afferents) and vascular components. All of these elements are connected within the fascia and they are responsible for the normal movement of the joint. Since the brain is responsible for a motor direction rather than movement of specific muscles, it must depend upon the MFUs to provide the necessary information to allow the body to function in a unified coordinated manner. Brains only interpret the movement patterns and changes in directions. In the motor cortex, entire areas are controlled (eg, hands, lips, or legs). This point is critical for the understanding of motor function. The muscles function by way of MFUs as they move in different directions and in various ways (Stecco, 2004; Stecco, 2009).

To explain different dysfunctions we need terms and language that our brains can understand. Luigi invented the idea of segments and MFUs to explain the body in an easier way and find the impaired movement in a more specific way. Based on some of the above information, for ease of analysis, Luigi proposed the idea of relating 14 body segments (eg, neck, scapula, and shoulder) to their specific MFUs. Each segment is composed of six MFUs representing the six directions of motion along three anatomic planes (Fig. 1.4).

In his second book, *Pain and the Neuromyofascial Sequences* (1990), Luigi introduced the first FM treatment protocol: data collection, hypothesis, and verifications. During this time his interests in the internal or visceral dysfunctions were beginning. At the same time Luigi also united the aspect of motor verification to the FM. In order to correctly communicate the findings in motor verification, the classic terminologies of flexion and extension needed to be abandoned. He decided that it would be clearer to reference movement to the planes of space. For example, flexion of the hip is more clearly communicated as "antemotion

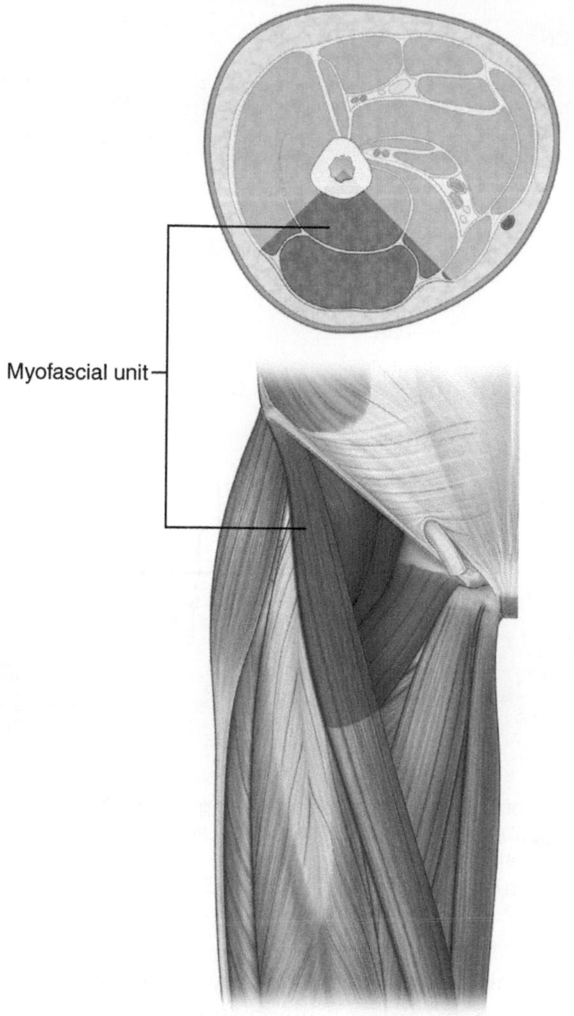

Fig. 1.3 One key element of fascial manipulation: the myofascial unit. The image area highlights the AN-CX; it is located on the anterior part of the thigh, inferior to the inguinal ligament, medial to the sartorius muscle. AN - forward movement, antemotion; CX - area of the hip.

or antepulsion of the hip" and extension of the knee as "antemotion or antepulsion of the knee."

In *La Manipolizione Neuroconnectivale* (1996), specific areas in the fascia of the MFU were identified. They are called centers of coordination (CC), which are points where FM treatment is performed. CC points are specified by the six movement directions ante (AN), retro (RE), lateral (LA), medial (ME), external rotation (ER), and internal rotation (IR) and by the segment. For example, RE-CL refers to the point that functions in the backward motion of the neck (CL=collum). Wisely, Luigi used Latin names for the segments (eg, coxa/

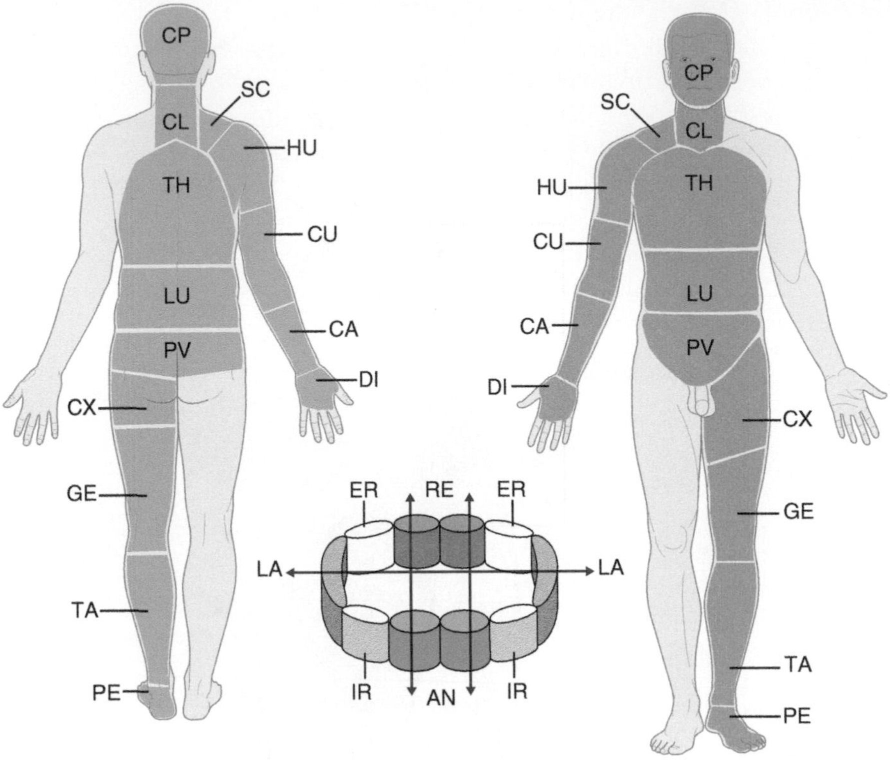

Fig. 1.4 Overall picture of the segments used in fascial manipulation. CP - head; CL - neck; TH - thorax; LU - lumbar area; PV - pelvic area; CX - hip; GE - knee; TA - shin; PE - foot; SC - area of shoulder girdle; HU - area of glenohumeral joint; CU - arm; CA - forearm; DI - hand; AN - forward motion; RE - backward motion; LA - lateral flexion or abduction; ME - adduction; ER - external rotation; IR - internal rotation.

hip, genu/knee), allowing communication by practitioners worldwide. By this sort of identifier (motion/location), points are named in every segment of the body. For example AN-CX would indicate the point controlling forward movement in the hip area (Table 1.2).

The CC is the site where unidirectional forces or muscular vectors converge. It is located between the deep fascia layers and it coordinates the action of unidirectional monoarticular and biarticular muscle fibers. It is the point where the vector forces act in the area of each MFU. Usually distal to the CC is found the center

TABLE 1.2 ■ **Movement Directions in Sagittal, Frontal, and Horizontal Planes**

Sagittal Plane	Frontal Plane	Horizontal Plane
Antemotion (AN)	Lateromotion (LA)	Extrarotation (ER)
Retromotion (RE)	Mediomotion (ME)	Intrarotation (IR)

of perception (CP), the site where movement occurring at the joint is perceived. Due to densification of the CC, the CP could become painful because of poor synchronization of the unidirectional forces of the MFU causing an inappropriate or excessive traction to the mechanoreceptors located in the CP area. Pain from the CC could be referred to the CP area. Functional passive, resisted, or active testing of the CP area could elicit pain (Fig. 1.5) (Stecco, 2004; Stecco, 2009).

After the release of his 1996 work, Luigi began to explore another set of points called the centers of fusion (CF). It was necessary to account for movement not only along the axes of the three planes, but also for complex and intermediate movements. These points were identified as junctions of the forces of three MFUs. For example, a CF such as antelateral (AN-LA) would synchronize the two MFUs and their respective CCs, AN and LA (Fig. 1.5). Associated with

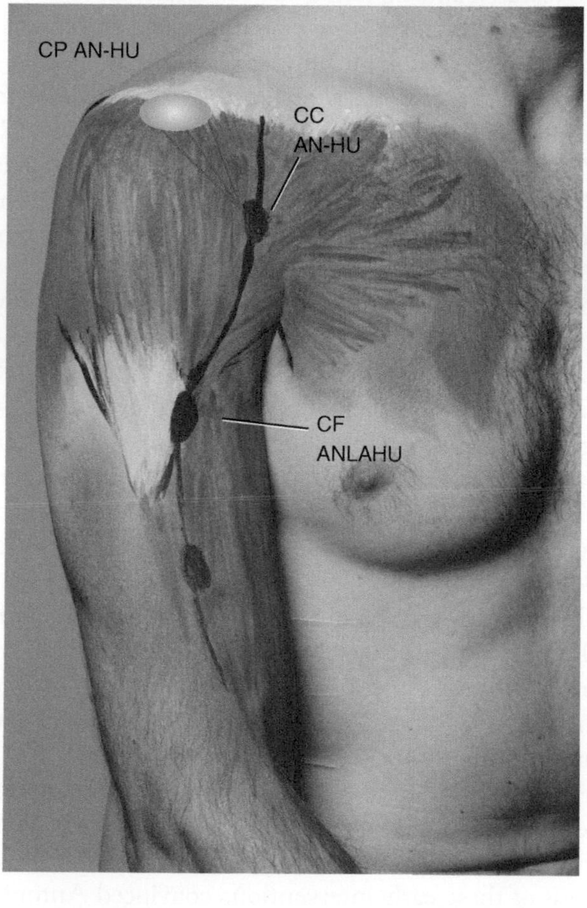

Fig. 1.5 Center of coordination (CC) and center of perception (CP) of AN-HU located in the anterior part of the deltoid. Center of fusion (CF) of AN-LA-HU located at the insertional area of deltoid muscle, anterior part. AN means movement forward; LA indicates lateral motion; HU is a location of the points in the arm.

the CFs is always a rotational MFU consisting of either ER or IR. CFs are located over retinaculas, periarticular structures (near joint tendons), and in the trunk along the lines of union of some muscles. They synchronize MFU activity by way of Golgi tendon organs. In contrast, CCs are associated with spindle cells. It was around the year 2002 that the older nomenclature of "neuroconnective manipulation" was changed to FM.

Luigi's enthusiasm for anatomy led him to become familiar with the works of Leonardo Da Vinci, who was an anatomist in addition to his other achievements, and Scarpa. Luigi appreciated some of the older descriptions, for example, of the deltoid muscle showing six compartments compared with modern texts showing three parts. He felt that the older renderings explained the deltoid's function more precisely (Fig. 1.6). Consequently, the Stecco concepts, emphasizing both functional and fascial research and exploring the continuity and connections of fascia to surrounding muscles and fascial layers, have helped to explain function (and dysfunction) in ways not possible in simpler present-day models.

In 2004, Luigi released a theoretical text, *Fascial Manipulation for Musculoskeletal Pain*, explaining the full nature of FM. This was followed in 2009 by *Fascial Manipulation Practical Part*, written by Luigi and his daughter Carla Stecco, MD, a Professor at Padua University. Books and studies are clarifying the background, basics, and meaning behind the CC and CF. This is the way to make FM powerful and accepted.

Carla Stecco pursues anatomic dissection research to this day, focusing on revealing the exact nature of the fascial layers, their connections, and orientations. In these studies, she collaborates with the Anatomy Faculties of René Descartes University in Paris, France, and the University of Padua in Italy, where she is an orthopedic surgeon and a professor of anatomy. Carla, the elder of two children, was educated early in fascial research by her father. It can be stated that she was "born in fascia." Although she was very interested, she was not completely convinced of the value of her father's work until she entered medical school. Some of the things she knew to be true were not viewed as factual, or even important, by other doctors. In fact, the very basic texts sometimes had incorrect or unclear information. She was convinced her father was on the right track and focused all her research on extending the knowledge of the fascia. One of her goals is to strengthen the scientific background for FM. Her dream is to gather a powerful team, which can do research in the field of fascia (Fig. 1.7).

Luigi's son Antonio graduated as a physiatrist. Antonio was an active athlete who suffered from recurrent minor traumas. Fortunately, he had a father who was on the spot to treat him with manual therapy based on his growing knowledge of fascia. The success of these early interventions convinced Antonio, once he had completed his MD degree, to continue studying physical medicine and rehabilitation. He has become a fellow in ultrasonography for musculoskeletal dysfunction and has also earned a PhD in sports medicine. In collaboration with

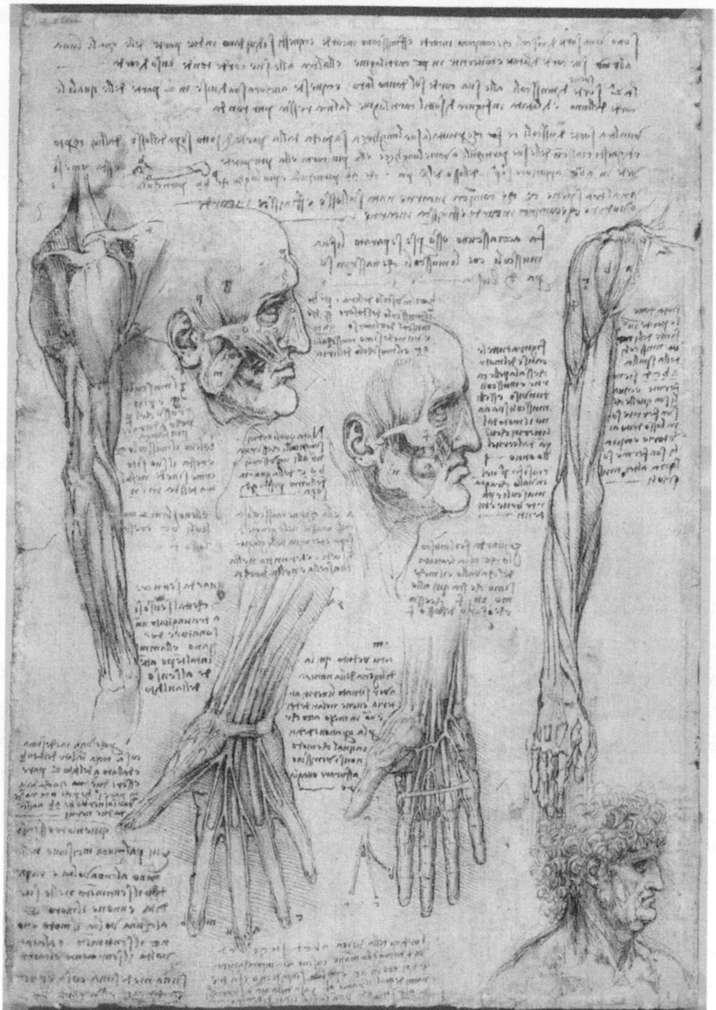

Fig. 1.6 Leonardo Da Vinci's idea of deltoid muscle (1508–1510, the six studies of the bones and the muscles of the arm). Royal Collection Trust, © Her Majesty Queen Elizabeth II 2016.

colleagues at Touro University in New York, NY, he continues to research both the mechanical and clinical aspects of manual therapies. One of Antonio's major contributions to the field of fascial research has been the description of the increase of fascial stiffness due to modification of the viscosity of the hyaluronic acid between the layers of collagen fibers in the deep fascia. An increase of viscosity alters the dynamic response of the mechanoreceptors embedded in the fascia. It is considered to be one of the mechanisms of the myofascial pain syndrome. Antonio, like his sister, has a passion for continuing work on the scientific

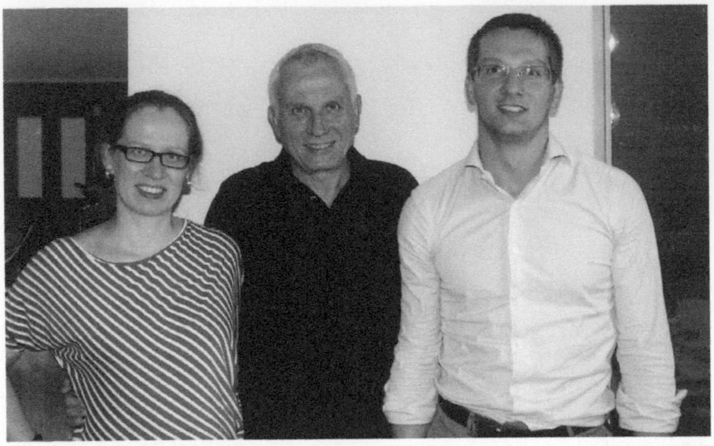

Fig. 1.7 Carla, Antonio, and Luigi Stecco.

background of FM. In addition, he circles the globe teaching other orthopedic clinicians the now extensive diagnosis and treatment methods of FM.

Luigi continues the work of development and exploration with his family (Fig. 1.8). He is currently writing the results of his clinical use of treating the visceral fascia using the same treatment techniques that FM has found successful in restoring musculoskeletal function. He is also exploring the psychological aspects of the body and its connections to fascia: psychosomatic effects. Dysfunction, not pathology, is his focus. As tension is transmitted via the fascial system, his work centers around the relationship of tension and the psychological system. Psychogenic factors can play a part in fascial connection within apparatus, systems, catenary, tensile structures, and superficial fascia. Alesandro Lowan and William Dryke have done research into this fascinating area and Luigi is intent on furthering their efforts. The fascial-psychological connection has yet to be fully understood and Luigi is approaching the work with his usual thoroughness. It has been demonstrated that somatic problems can have psychological effects, and the reverse is also true. Luigi has a sparkle in his eyes when he is speaking about fascia and its connections to the body. Fascia can be referred to as a never-ending web, and, likewise, the development of FM is a process that will never end. The enthusiasm will keep the ideas fresh and will widen the perspective of manual therapy and its possibilities.

Both Carla and Antonio continue to research the aspects of the fascial system in addition to presenting research and treatment strategies to professional groups throughout the world. They and other researchers continue to study and publish, furthering the understanding of the fascial system and centers of coordination and fusion. FM is now widely accepted as an effective treatment modality and learning of the characteristics and function of the fascial system has advanced substantially

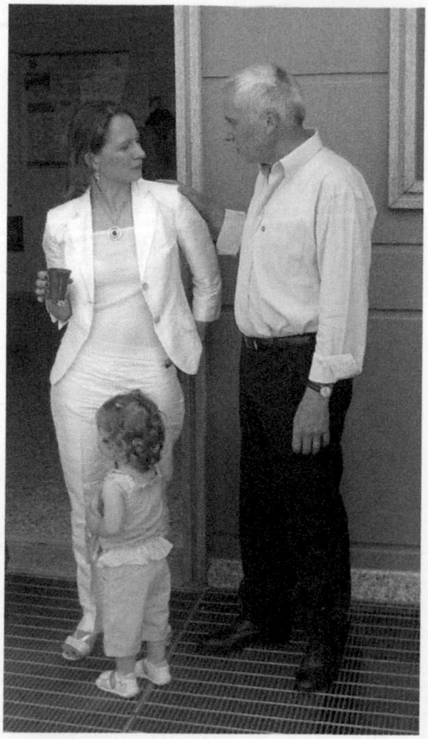

Fig. 1.8 Carla and Luigi after a fascial manipulation course in front of the Stecco Medical Center, Thiene, Italy.

from the early days. Carla's dream is to gather a powerful research team so that the fascial system can be understood as deeply as the other anatomic systems are. She devotes her professional research to understanding and proving the anatomic and histologic properties of fascial tissue. She uses dissection, microscopic, and electron microscopic studies, as well as other research techniques, to advance understanding. Her most recent textbook, *Functional Atlas of the Human Fascial System*, published by Elsevier in 2015, represents a revolution in the history of anatomy. As her professor, Raffaele De Caro, writes in the foreword, "This Atlas is the first accurate description of the human fasciae. It has revived the use of the scientific method for the study of human anatomy." (Fig. 1.9).

Luigi still practices and is always eager to follow the progress of patients he treats with FM. His fame has spread and patients regularly travel long distances to see him. It is not unusual for a patient to report that a problem of some years' duration has been resolved in fairly short order with FM. Luigi has the practiced eye to see the origin of the problem and the hands to resolve it. Quite often the patients' stories are complicated and have many aspects. Successful outcomes are keeping him inspired and he still has the enthusiasm to learn and develop FM further (Interview of Carla Stecco and Luigi Stecco, 2013).

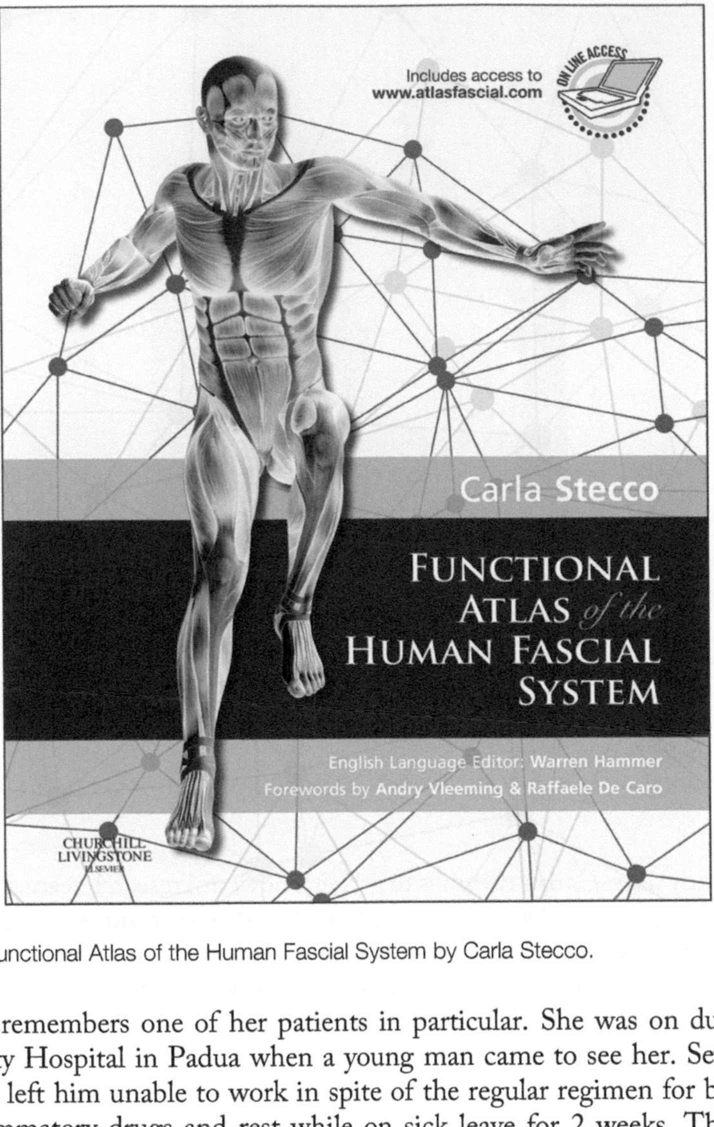

Fig. 1.9 Functional Atlas of the Human Fascial System by Carla Stecco.

Carla remembers one of her patients in particular. She was on duty in the University Hospital in Padua when a young man came to see her. Severe back pain had left him unable to work in spite of the regular regimen for back pain: antiinflammatory drugs and rest while on sick leave for 2 weeks. The patient was crying and said that he couldn't afford to continue to take sick leave. She treated him with FM and he was pain free when he left her office. As he hugged her in gratitude, she realized very personally how powerful FM was. She had just received very real proof of its effectiveness. Scientific studies are necessary, but the sincere gratitude in one patient's eyes was enough to convince her that if resolving such acute pain was possible by identifying the correct points and treating them, she would do it (Interview of Carla Stecco and Luigi Stecco, 2013) (see Video 2).

Antonio enjoys teaching and he remembers one man from São Paulo, Brazil, who was not able to bend forward at all without pain. Actually, every movement direction was painful when he did movement verification. While teaching, having cases during the course is always exciting. Expectations and interests of the participants and people who are coming to have a treatment in front of the audience challenge everybody. In this particular case, Antonio managed to solve the movement dysfunction and the man was able to bend forward without pain. Also other movements of the back were pain free. These moments are the highlights of teaching and spread the idea of FM further.

Using dissections and anatomic studies, the Stecco family continues to improve and amplify the combination of movement testing and palpatory verification of points responsible for fascial dysfunction. It is crucial for the therapist to understand how to palpate correctly to identify the points to treat. This requires an in-depth understanding of anatomy (Fig. 1.10). The manual treatment technique is fairly easy to master, but identifying the points upon which to apply it requires an advanced understanding of the biomechanical model of the human body and the functional meaning of this model. This is why the method can be successfully used only after diligent study and training. A trained therapist should be able to choose what technique to use to help the patient the most. The timing and duration of the treatment can only be optimized with practice and study. The therapist should respect the first teaching of Hippocrates (460 BC): *primum, non nocere* (first, do no harm). The results of FM should be immediate and there should be visible results after the first visit.

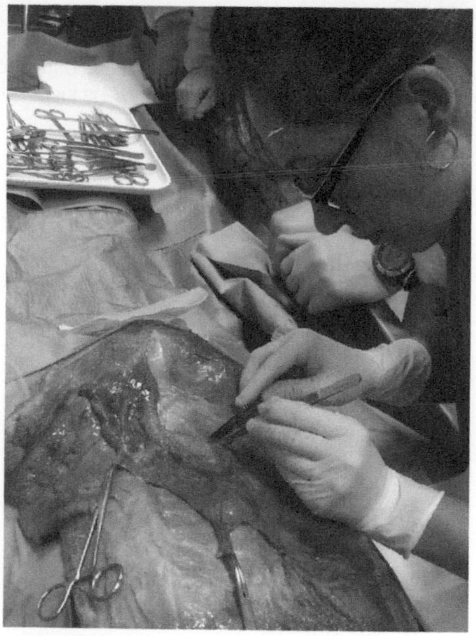

Fig. 1.10 Carla performing a dissection in Padua University.

FM is now known and recognized by its logo. Scapulas and a vertebral column are entwined by the two snakes of the caduceus, the symbol of medicine. The L and S incorporated unobtrusively in the logo are Luigi's initials as a recognition of his pioneering work (Fig. 1.11).

FM is now taught in 40 countries and, at present, approximately 1000 new clinicians receive training every year (Fig. 1.12). The very first teachers of FM were Ergole Borgini, Andrea Turrina, Mirco Branchini, Julie Ann Day, Luca Ramilli, Giorgio Rucli, and Lorenzo Copetti. All teachers are now trained and certified by the Fascial Manipulation Association (AMF), established in 2008 (Fig. 1.13). It is a not-for-profit organization founded to unite all professionals who work for the improvement and diffusion of FM. The AMF also promotes

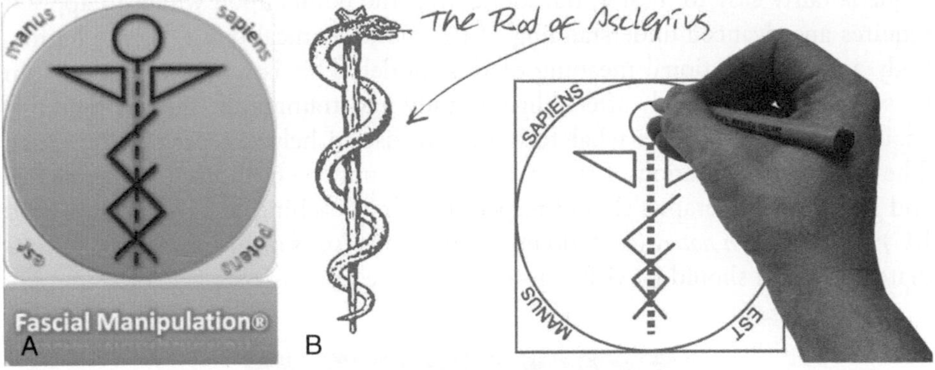

Fig. 1.11 The fascial manipulation logo—*Manus sapiens, potens est.* Shoulder blades and vertebral column are combined with Luigi's initials L and S. The figure is inspired by the rod of Asclepius.

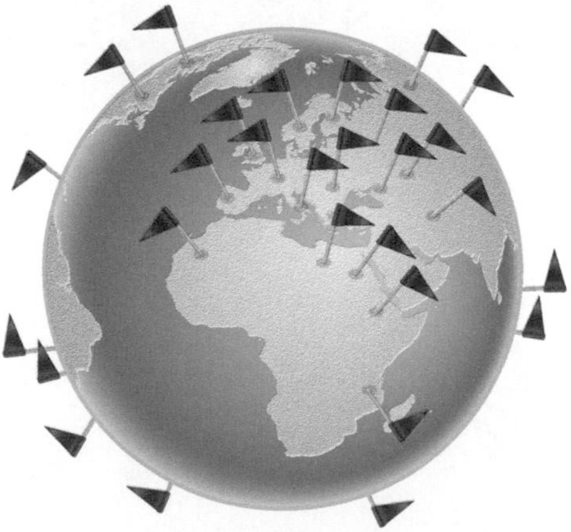

Fig. 1.12 Fascial manipulation spreads all over the world. The FM courses are taught in many countries by educated teachers.

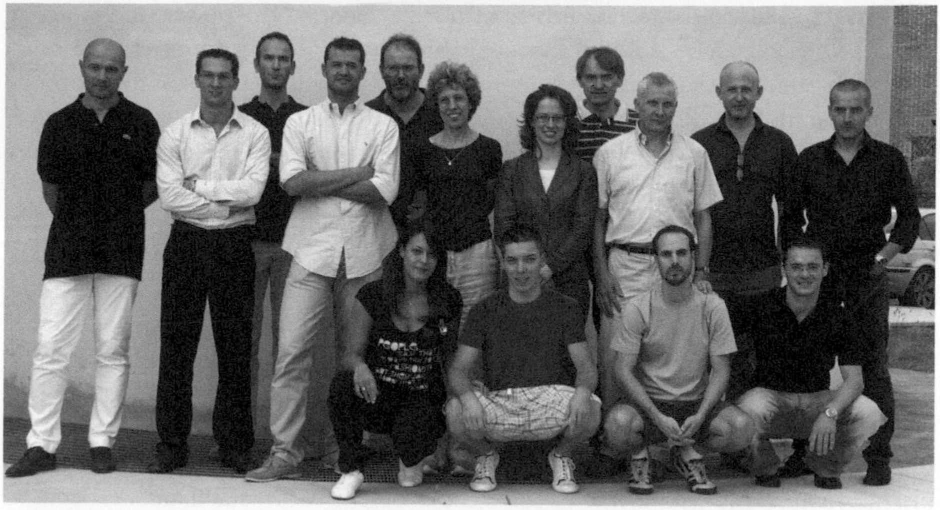

Fig. 1.13 The first fascial manipulation teachers. The method started in Italy and the first teachers were Italians.

and supports research in the field of pain relief, anatomy, and physiopathology of the fascia, fascial pain, and pain linked to internal fasciae. Its goal is to provide the scientific groundwork for all methods and theories dealing with the role of the fascia in musculoskeletal and internal dysfunction in living beings, in addition to various pathologies as yet unsupported by adequate scientific understanding. Thus, ultimately, it is to benefit people afflicted by such pathologies (Fig. 1.14).

Fig. 1.14 The Fascial Manipulation Association logo. AMF is a not-for-profit organization and it is founded to unite all FM professionals.

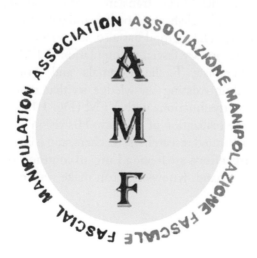

Many FM teachers have had their own experience of the power of "knowing hands" when they have suffered from pain and dysfunction syndromes. A case in point is Stefano Casadei, physiotherapist, who was a tennis player active in tournaments in his 20s. Elbow pain forced him off the courts and he sought help from so many professionals that he had almost lost hope when he arrived at Luigi Stecco's clinic. Not only did Luigi relieve the elbow pain, but in Stefano he recognized the spark of enthusiasm for FM work. Stefano signed up for training in FM and has become one of the teachers travelling from country to country teaching this remarkable method. He says he is very enthusiastic about seeking and finding just the right treatment for patients. It is impossible to get bored, Stefano asserts, because every patient is unique and you must discover the relevant parts of the patient's history to understand how the pain developed. If you do not understand this, treatment of random points will be to no avail. There is no specific protocol to obey, as every patient is different, and you have to respect his/her history and find a way to solve the problem with your hands.

FM texts (the practical and the theoretical) are generally the starting point of all training in FM. The third book of the series deals with the diagnoses and treatment of dysfunction in the visceral fascia. This book, originally published in 2013, was coauthored by Luigi and Carla Stecco. All three of these books were translated into English by Julie Ann Day, who is herself an experienced teacher of FM. She has also been active in teaching internationally and lecturing to congresses on FM research. She is the "go to" person when a practitioner anywhere in the world has a question about the method—she is always willing to help. The series of FM books was expanded with Luigi's *Atlante di Fisiologia della Fascia Muscolare* published in 2015.

The FM texts have now been translated into Japanese, Korean, Polish, Finnish, German, Italian, English, and Spanish and will shortly be translated into Portuguese and Chinese. The method has also been extended to members of the animal kingdom and veterinary fascial manipulation (VFM) is being developed by Finnish physiotherapists Tuulia Luomala and Mika Pihlman. These researchers are extending existing knowledge so that many types of animals may receive relief from dysfunctions with VFM (Fig. 1.15) (see Video 3).

For Luigi, FM is the realization of a dream. His vision is now being enlarged and spread by many dedicated researchers, teachers, and clinicians throughout the world. These wonderful efforts are freeing Luigi to continue to explore the potential of the power of the hand. Knowledge can make you free.

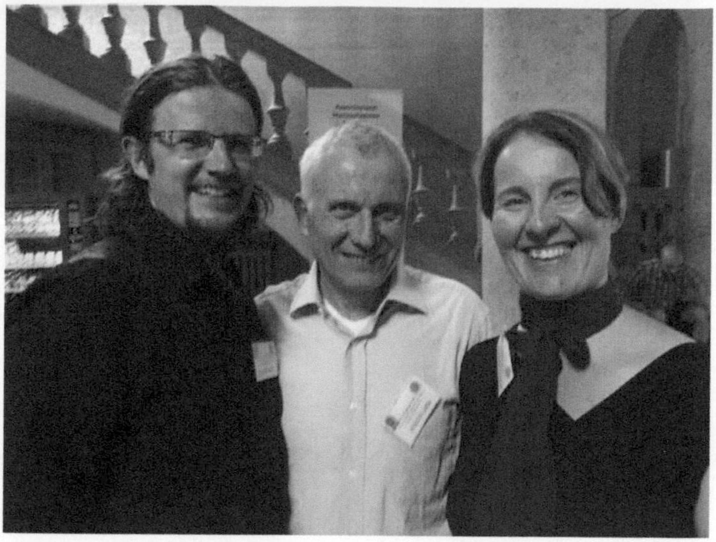

Fig. 1.15 Mika, Luigi, and Tuulia participating in the annual AMF congress.

References

Interview of Carla Stecco and Luigi Stecco, Stecco Medical Centrum, Zugliano, Italy, September 14, 2013.

Stecco, L., 2004. Fascial Manipulation for Musculoskeletal Pain. Piccin, Padua, Italy.

Stecco, L., Stecco, C., 2009. Fascial Manipulation Practical Part. Piccin, Padua, Italy.

CHAPTER 2

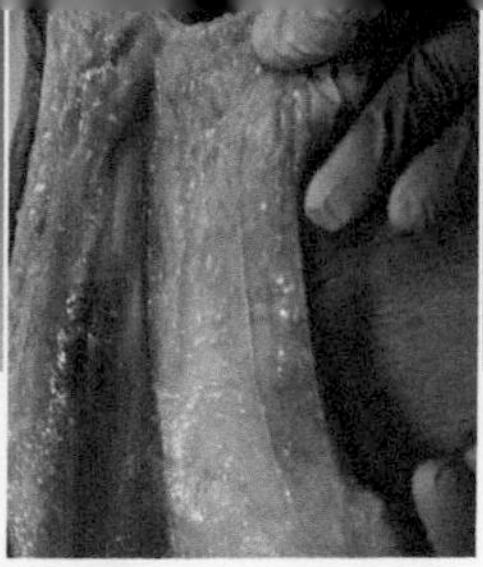

Anatomy of the Fascia from the Clinical Point of View

The pivotal role of the fascial system in maintaining the proper function of the human body is being increasingly recognized by professionals who regularly treat soft tissue problems. This includes doctors, therapists, and sports trainers among others. Knowledge of the fascial system's characteristics and functions is rapidly spreading from primary medical researchers to professionals in many health fields throughout the world. Understanding fascial function can even change the way people exercise in a gym, especially with regard to their workout regimen. Trainers are recommending foam rolling and stretching routines based on new fascial knowledge. People involved in dance, yoga, Pilates, and martial arts are able to improve performance safety using the discoveries of fascial organization and function. Therapists in many areas are developing techniques to modify fascia and integrate it into treatment regimes. Both superficial and deep fascia within the body can be treated with manual methods directly or indirectly and also with instrument-assisted modalities. Surgeons are beginning to take connective tissue into account as an integral part of surgical procedures in order to promote wound healing, scar reduction, and tissue restoration and to minimize damage to veins, nerves, and muscles embedded in fascia. Now that fascial anatomy has been researched thoroughly, this knowledge must be integrated into our fundamental understanding of human anatomy. Anatomists are slowly beginning to realize that the fascia is not just a covering; it is actually a sensory organ that is responsible for proprioception and bodily communication (Fig. 2.1).

The corpus of knowledge of the fascial system has been growing at an astonishingly rapid rate. At present, approximately 1000 peer-reviewed studies are published annually. Adding explanatory articles and internet blogs, the total amounts easily to several thousand per year (Fig. 2.2). Actually fascial research is not new, since peer-reviewed studies have been published with some frequency since the late 1960s. Prior to this upsurge, the founder of osteopathic manual medicine, A.T. Still (1828–1917) wrote about fascia and its treatment in the late 1890s (Still, 1899). Ancient Chinese writings described meridians laying approximately 1 cm under the skin (more superficial than acupuncture meridians). These meridians, termed "muscle sinews," were broader than the acupuncture meridians.

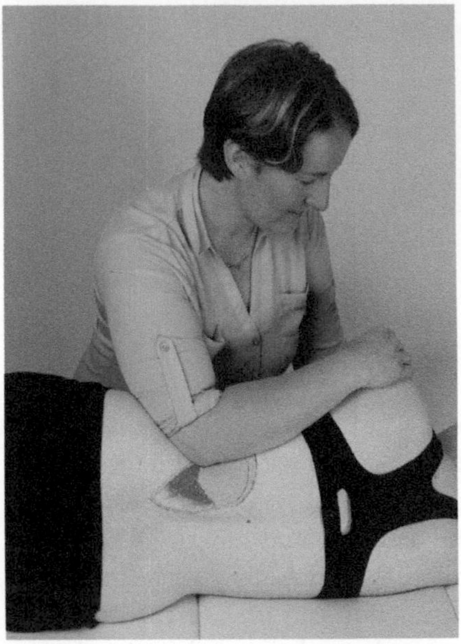

Fig. 2.1 Fascial manipulation treatment combined with anatomic thinking. Therapist should feel the fascial layers under the fingers or elbow and understand the fascial anatomy.

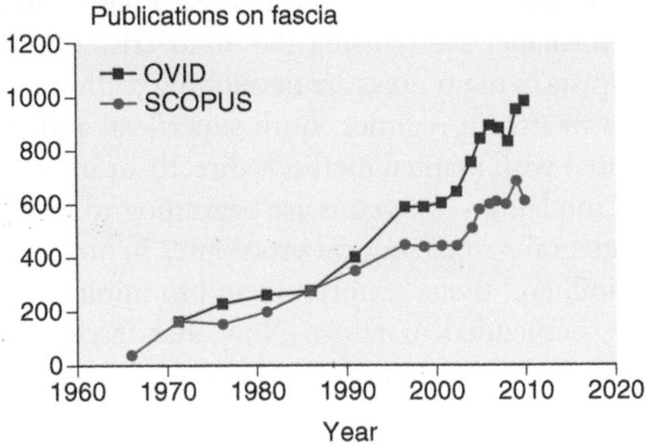

Fig. 2.2 Growth of studies concerning fascia.

The Chinese looked at human anatomy from a different perspective than their Western colleagues. They described in careful detail nerve continua as well as vein continua, but they did not focus on single muscles. Rather they envisaged subcutaneous anatomy as an arrangement of longitudinal channels, or "sinews."

Western medicine has focused on specific segments in isolation. Shoulder problems, for example, are analysed and treated based on current knowledge of the shoulder only. Pain in the knee is analysed as a localized lesion. The fascial system as a unifying and connecting structure was rarely examined. In the 1850s, Jacob and Bourgery's *Anatomy* showed the epimysium and deep and superficial fascia very clearly. The text used diagrams to portray the fascia—without muscles in some areas (Fig. 2.3). Testut (1895) and Chiarugi and Bucciante (1975) also wrote anatomy texts that included some analysis of fascia. The majority of anatomy researchers treated fascia as connective tissue only. This tissue served only to fill the empty spaces around more interesting and important tissues. Thus fascial tissue in contemporary anatomic studies is not new but rather finally understood as a functioning and important kinetic system (Jacob and Bourgery, 1850; Schleip et al., 2012).

After Jacob's and Still's work, the next wave of researchers seriously interested in the fascia emerged around 1940 when Mézières, Rolf, Travell, and Simons published their work. Then, in the 1980s, Busquet, Struyf-Denys, Souchard, and Stecco started to develop their ideas on fascial treatment. Each researcher added to the knowledge base with the objective of developing more effective diagnosis and treatment methods. Every method has its own theoretical base, but the differences between them has been narrowing and with this coming together, there has been an increasing recognition of the connections between the fascial sequences that can lead to more precise analysis and treatment. Understanding interconnected tensional complexes is the focus of the new treatments

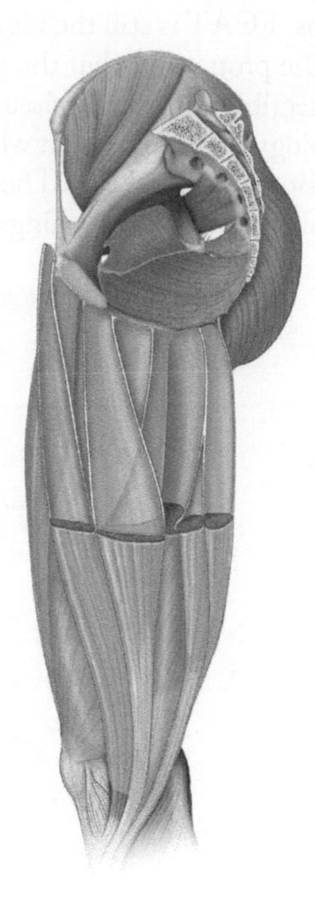

Fig. 2.3 Anatomy of the thigh without muscles inside the fascia.

(Fig. 2.4). Carla Stecco's seminal work, *Functional Atlas of the Human Fascial System* (2015), has clearly laid out fascial anatomy for the first time and proposed a rational nomenclature for the use of practitioners and researchers alike. Histologic and anatomic studies provide the basis for fascial manipulation (FM).

History of the Nomenclature

In 1983, the International Anatomical Nomenclature Committee developed a classification system for all connective tissue structures. This nomenclature includes superficial and deep fascia. All soft tissues under the skin (including fat cells and fat lobules) were classified as superficial fascia. In the abdomen, superficial fascia was, in turn, divided into two types: an adipose layer (more fat cells than membrane) named after Camper; and a membranous layer (more membrane than fat cells) called Scarpa's fascia. Under the superficial fascia lay deep fascia, the fascia profundus. It is denser and firmer tissue than superficial fascia. Researchers are hampered somewhat by terminology that is not standardized (Schleip et al., 2012; Stecco C., 2015b).

In 1998, the Federative Committee on Anatomical Terminology (FCAT, 1998) proposed different terms. FCAT is still the highest authority on nomenclature of the anatomic terms. The proposal is that the fascia should be described as "sheaths, sheets" or other dissectible connective tissue aggregations. This diverse and nonstandardized terminology was still present when the first Fascia Research Congress was held in 2007 in Boston, MA, USA. There, researchers and clinicians convened for the purpose of, among other things, creating an agreed-upon

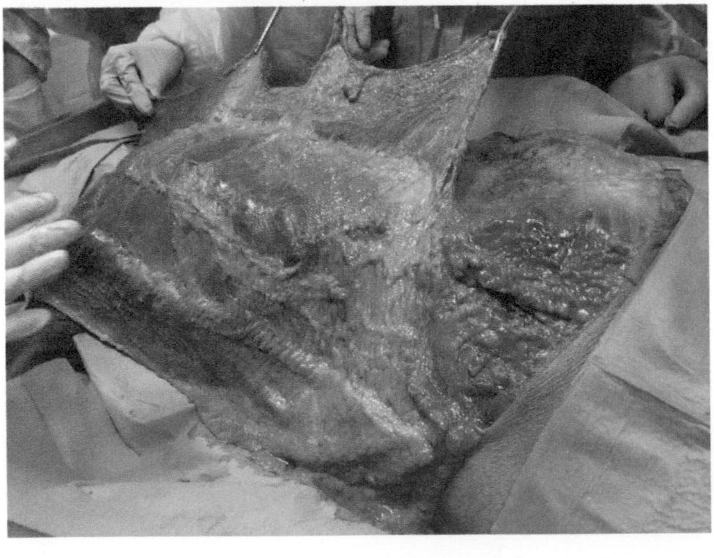

Fig. 2.4 Dissection image from the fascial system of the back.

common terminology. This was the starting point of a scientific fascial community, uniting different professionals and researchers. The need for fascial research and tests was apparent and the Congress decided to convene every third year to review the latest research in this relatively new domain. The Congress has grown and has been quite successful, building on the strengths of this first session.

In September 2015 in Washington, DC, USA, the 4th Fascia Research Congress was held. Many different opinions were expressed. Leading fascial researchers and clinicians presented and discussed the newest research in their areas of interest. Professor Carla Stecco from the University of Padua, Italy, presented her extensive work on mapping the entire fascial system. A working definition of the fascia was agreed upon: "Fascia is a sheath, a sheet or any number of other dissectible aggregations of connective tissue that forms beneath the skin to attach, enclose, separate muscles and internal organs." A more general and functional definition includes the role of the fascia: Fascia interacts, connects, and permits communication among its different elements so that an interdependent complex called the fascial system is formed. Research groups are now making substantial progress towards the goal of creating new and useful fascial terminology. The new terminology will include both anatomic and functional aspects of the fascia (Stecco C., 2015b; Stecco and Schleip, 2015) (Fig. 2.5).

To understand the function and architecture of the fascial system, it is important to understand its composition. Fascia must be understood first and foremost as connective tissue (textus connectivus) (FCAT, 1998). Carla Stecco's *Functional Atlas of the Human Fascial System* (2015) highlights the importance of fascia. This text is the first anatomic atlas analysing fascial connection and

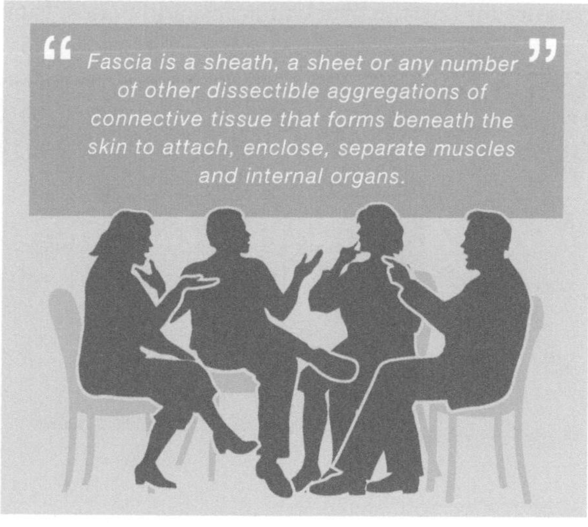

Fig. 2.5 Group of researchers working toward consensus on the terminology.

composition. It is not a simple task to clarify the meaning of fascia and its architecture. Attempts to define fascia in a single word are doomed to failure, like calling a nut and a watermelon the same thing. The fascial system is complex with composition, orientation, and functions that vary widely. That's why we need precise descriptive terms to communicate useful meaning in both an anatomical and functional way.

From the clinical point of view as well, we need specific terms. What precisely are we manipulating when treating a patient? And how do we refer to the different layers? The first contact will always be the skin. It is a sensitive structure incorporating many receptors that react to temperature, stretching, pressure, and tactile changes. Hearing, olfactory, vision, or taste perception may be lost, but we can adapt and survive. However, loss of sense of touch is serious and almost impossible to compensate for. We use touch-sensory vocabulary to describe things perceived with the other senses. For instance, "I get a kick out of good music." The sense of touch is fundamental in the connection of our mind and body (Fig. 2.6). These interesting connections are useful when combining clinical and theoretical knowledge. What we need first is a commonly understood vocabulary, so that fascial knowledge can be shared, studied, and properly understood.

What is Connective Tissue?

Connective tissue (CT) can be thought of as a key link of the locomotor and visceral system. The CT holds everything together, that is to say it connects them. Every single cell, from muscle to nerve and from bone to skin is surrounded by some kind of CT. This tissue holds those single cells together to form more complex tissues, such as organs (eg, the liver), muscles, and bones. Interstices between

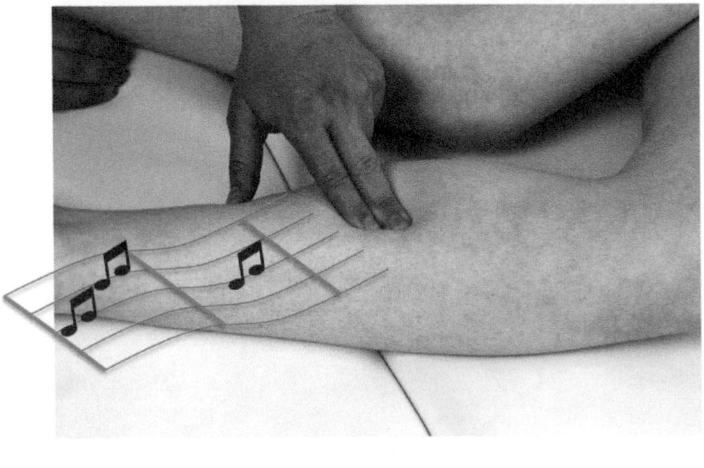

Fig. 2.6 Image of palpation and its connection to the tissue and the feeling hands.

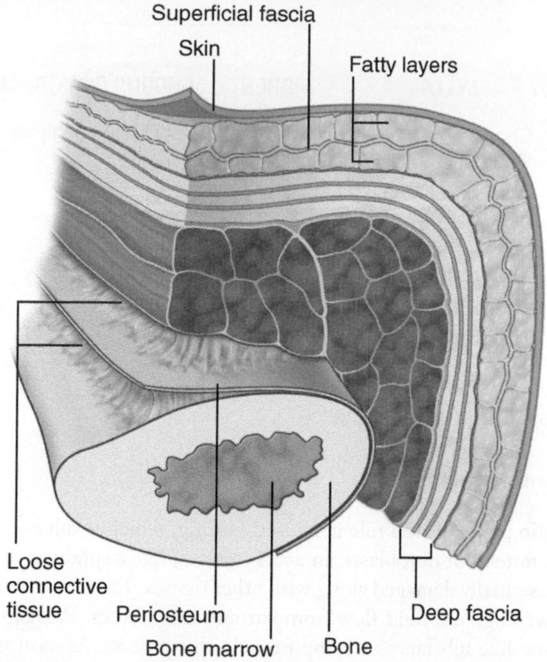

Fig. 2.7 Image of fascial layers and anatomy from skin to bone.

tissues are filled with CT forming a looser and more flexible environment for the tissues. Quite simply, CT exists everywhere in the body, forming a three-dimensional network in layers of various sizes like a "never-ending web" (Fig. 2.7). The basic composition of connective tissue has three components: cells, fibres, and ground substance.

THE CELLS

The cells (Fig. 2.8) provide the metabolic properties of biological tissue, which means they are responsible for all vital functions of our body. Fibroblasts are the most common cell type in the human tissue and in fact in all animal tissue. They are the building blocks of the body. Collagen fibres and other intercellular materials (like glycosaminoglycans, or GAGs, as discussed later) are produced by fibroblasts. Cells react also to stretch, compression, torque, and shear. Deformation (via touch) can modify the process of cell organization. Fascial work can operate at different depths, directions, and force based on what the patient needs as revealed in diagnosis. Meltzer et al. (2010) proposed that fascial stimulation through gentle massage may speed up the recovery process of tissues. On the other hand, excessively vigorous techniques will slow down repair of tissues (Box 2.1).

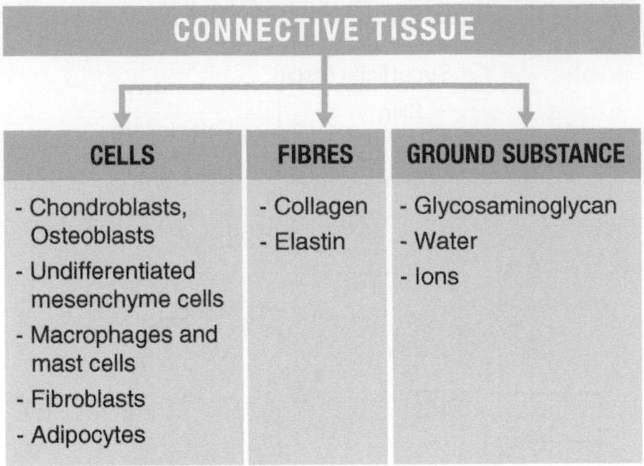

Fig. 2.8 Cells, fibres, and ground substance.

BOX 2.1 Wound Healing

The fibroblasts also play a critical role in wound healing, which involves stimulation of fibrocytes that induce mitosis of fibroblasts. In acute injuries, like a sprain in the calf muscle, connective tissue is essentially damaged along with other tissues. The inflammatory process begins after bleeding, swelling, and fluid flow from surrounding tissues. Prostaglandin, bradykinin, and other hormone-like substances are important in this process. As soon as the inflammation lessens, the fibroblasts gather into the wounded area where they promote tissue regeneration (Butler, 2000; Stecco C., 2015a) (Fig. 2.9).

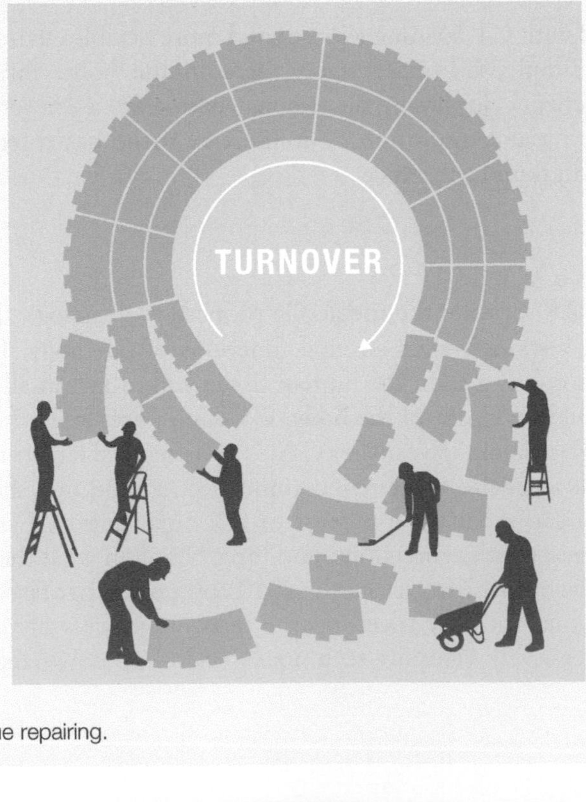

Fig. 2.9 Tissue repairing.

Adipocytes (adipose or fat cells) are found in the CT. Fat cells can also be stored in internal organs where they are called visceral fat. The adipose cells can be divided into white (unilocular cells) and brown fat cells (multilocular cells). Adipose cells in the subcutaneous tissue adhere tightly to a rich collagen mat also known as the membranous layer of the superficial fascia. Overall, fat cells store energy and they are extremely important for insulation (Drake et al., 2015; Stecco C., 2015a).

THE FIBRES

The fibres provide the mechanical properties of CT. They create the form of the tissue by giving strength to surrounding CT. Endomysium is a cover that surrounds the muscle cell. It is formed by fibroblasts. The fibres also have the power to transfer force generated by muscle cells, and they seem to get stronger and thicker when tensional stress is applied (Magnusson et al., 2010; Schleip and Müller, 2012). There are two types of fibres in CT: collagen fibres and elastic fibres. The collagen fibres are flexible, but only within the range of their tensile strength. To date, 28 different types of collagen have been identified and described. Collagen is the main structural protein in CT, making up approximately 35% of the whole-body protein content of the human body (Box 2.2). Almost 90% of the collagen of the muscles can be found in the perimysium (perimysium is CT surrounding bundles of muscle cells, or fasciculi) (McCormick, 1994; Müller, 2003).

Collagen fibres/fibrils usually align along the main lines of a mechanical load, but under pathological circumstances collagen fibrils can get very dense and may form cross-links. This can create dysfunction and compromise normal tissue response. A collagen fibre's lifespan varies depending on collagen types. To describe the length of the life of a collagen fibre, researchers use the term turnover time to indicate a biogeochemical cycle. It is a measure of how long it takes to fill or empty a particular nutrient reservoir. The human collagen turnover time has been estimated to be from 300 to 500 days. In animal studies, the rate differs.

BOX 2.2

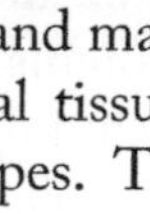

The word *collagen* comes from the Greek κόλλα (*kólla*), meaning "glue" and suffix -γέν, *-gen*, denoting "producing." The four most common types of collagen are:

- Type I: The most common type (90% of net amount in human body). It is found in skin, tendon, fascia, organ capsule, and bone.
- Type II: Mostly found in cartilage tissue.
- Type III: Also called reticular fibres, commonly found alongside type I. It can be found in loose connective tissue and around adipocytes.
- Type IV: Forms basal lamina of the epithelium. It more weblike than a regularly orientated fibril.

For instance, rat collagen fibre turnover time varies even more: intestine 20 days, liver 30 days, muscles 50 days, and tendons 110 days (Gerber, 1960). The metabolism of the rat is much faster than the human (estimated 7–10 times faster). Therefore those findings are not directly comparable with findings in human subjects (Carano and Sicialini, 1996; Stecco C., 2015a).

Elastin fibres are thinner than collagen fibres and they create a three-dimensional network around collagen fibres. Elastin is a protein that gives collagen the ability to tolerate stretch and distension. Elastin fibres and collagen fibres are not parallel. They lie across one another and/or spiral around one another so that they form a three-dimensional interacting superstructure, which gives final strength and elasticity to the whole tissue matrix (Kannus, 2008; Stecco C., 2015a). FM creates a mechanical load on CT in a particular way so that practitioners actually modify collagen and elastin fibres. This becomes a part of the continuing process of cell renewal in the body. The process continually alters cells, and practitioners essentially become an agent in this transformation by touch (mechanical load). Trauma, overuse, or misuse of the body also affects the fibres, often in a dysfunctional way, creating abnormal patterns of stress transmitted to the fibres.

THE GROUND SUBSTANCE

The ground substance provides viscosity and plasticity to the tissues (as do collagen and elastin fibres). The ground substance is composed of water, extracellular proteins, GAGs, and proteoglycans. Ground substance itself is a gel-like material including extrafibrillar matrix, but no collagen or elastin fibres. In other words, the collagen and elastin fibres create the previously mentioned three-dimensional network and the ground substance surrounds and fills the empty spaces. The entity formed by ground substance and fibres is called the extracellular matrix (ECM).

Proteoglycans and GAGs interact with each other. GAGs are long-chained polysaccharides attached to a core protein of the proteoglycan. Seven different groups of GAGs have been identified: hyaluronan (HA), chondroitin-4-sulfate, chondroitin-6-sulfate, dermaten sulfate, keratin sulfate, heparin sulfate, and heparin. Extracellular proteins stabilize the aggregates of proteoglycans and together form a “bottle-brush-like” structure (Fig. 2.10). HA is the most common GAG in the loose CT. In fact, it is not a typical GAG, because there is no sulfate group and it has a very long and rigid construction. HA provides moisture for the skin and makes it possible for muscles, tendons, and fascia to move against one another. HA also participates in the wound-healing process. GAGs have a negative charge that attracts water in order to form a hydrated gel. This gel is responsible for turgidity and viscoelasticity, as well as controlling the diffusion of various metabolites (Schleip et al., 2012; Stecco C., 2015a).

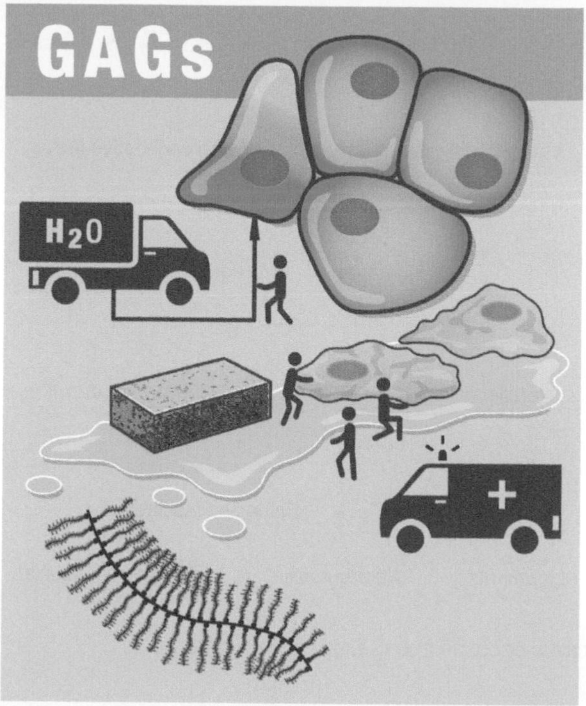

Fig. 2.10 Glycosaminoglycans (GAGs) viewed as a bottle-brush-like structure attracting the water inside the cells.

CLASSIFICATION OF CONNECTIVE TISSUE (see Video 4)

There are many types of CT, as mentioned earlier. CT can be divided into subgroups by density or regularity (Fig. 2.11). Loose connective tissue (LCT) and dense connective tissue (DCT) form two main groups. These two types of the connective tissue are closely connected both anatomically and functionally.

LCT, also known as areolar tissue, is the most common CT type. It is ubiquitous in the body, and is found between muscle cells, fascial layers, organs, veins, nerves, and other tissues. It has a twofold role of binding all tissues together, keeping them in place, and allowing tissues and layers to slide against each other (Fig. 2.12). In 2015, Jean-Claude Guimberteau, a French hand surgeon, made the first videos of living tissue by using small cameras inserted under the skin. His findings demonstrate both the importance of the LCT between fascial layers and the elasticity of this tissue (Guimberteau et al., 2015). The main cellular elements in LCT are fibroblasts and a few adipocytes. The adipocytes act as interstitial fillers that facilitate gliding potential. When adipocytes are organized in large lobules for storage purposes, they are commonly referred to as adipose tissue. Collagen is the most important fibril in LCT, although elastic fibres are also

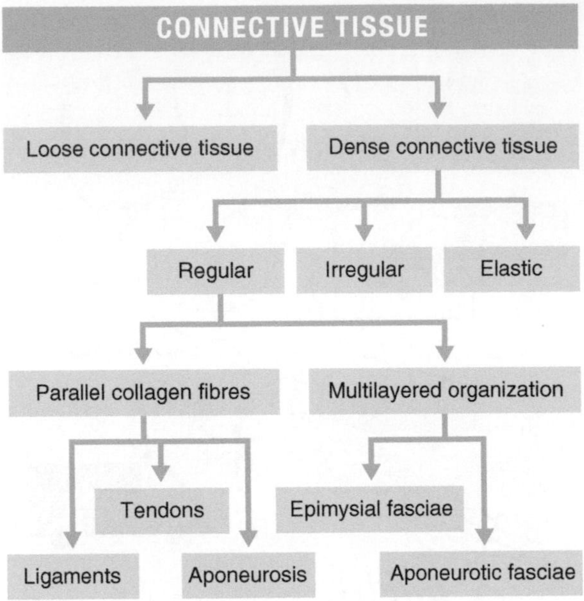

Fig. 2.11 Classification of connective tissue.

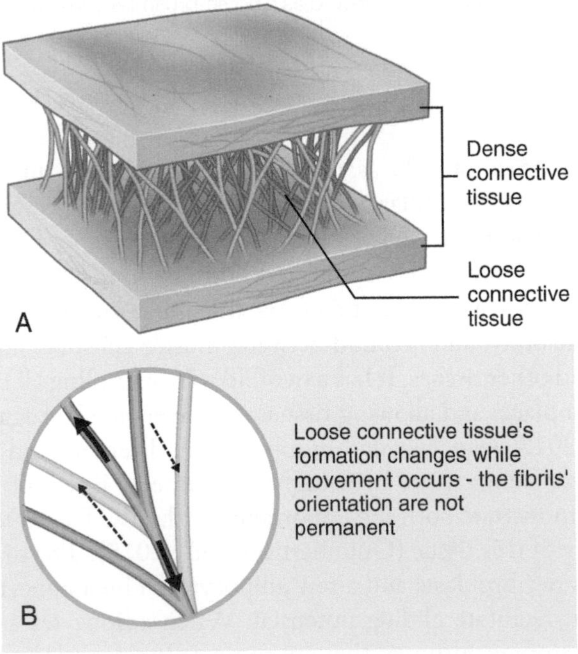

Fig. 2.12 Loose connective tissue is present everywhere between fascial layers and is the most common type of connective tissue.

present. Fibres extend in all directions, creating a loose network. LCT has a viscous, gel-like consistency depending on the interaction of GAGs, changes in pH level, and temperature (Stecco C., 2015a). Heat formed by cross-friction modifies the consistency of LCT.

Although mechanical properties are important, the ability of LCT to permit diffusion of oxygen, nutrients, and metabolites is vital. LCT is the initial site where antigens, bacteria, and other agents are identified and then destroyed. Further research is needed to identify and quantify the effect of the LCT on metabolites. According to Tom Findley's closing session at the 4th Fascia Research Congress in 2015, one of the future interests in the fascial research field will be metabolic issues, breathing, and their relationship with fascia.

DCT is a perfect matrix for force transmission over a distance and it creates anchors to help LCT hold tissues in place; for example, the sternopericardial ligament between the pericardium and the sternum. Overall, DCT is firm and strong with robust collagen fibres. Simplistically, more collagen results in firmer tissue. Collagen fibres in DCT are arranged parallel to one another to respond to mechanical load; for example, the Achilles tendon in the calf. Examples of DCT are tendons, ligaments, and deep fascia (Box 2.3). In the deep fascia, while there are parallel collagen fibres, there are other layers that have a different orientation of fibres. This type of structure allows the transmission of force in a variety of multidirectional planes (Benetazzo et al., 2011; Purslow, 2010). Moreover, mechanical load and tension increase collagen synthesis and make it more resistant to load stress. People who do heavy lifting and vigorous work throughout

BOX 2.3

Tractus iliotibialis, also known as the *iliotibial band (ITB)*, is an example of dense connective tissue. It runs from the ilium to the tibia as a bandlike structure. The anatomy of this structure is, however, not so simple. First, what is often depicted in anatomy texts differs from what anatomists observe in cadavers. True, it is a longitudinal form of DCT running along the lateral side of the thigh, but actually the ITB is a thickening of the deep fascia of the thigh area known as the fascia latae, and it is not bandlike. The fascia latae surrounds the whole thigh, not just the lateral side. Separating the so-called tractus from the fascia lata is possible only with a scalpel because they are part of the same structure (Stecco A. et al., 2013a). Second, and even more interesting, the tractus iliotibialis is not well developed or hardened in small children or persons who have used wheelchairs for several years. On the other hand, long distance runners, football players, and weightlifters seem to have a strong, clearly visible ITB. This indicates that the tractus iliotibialis becomes visible and therefore identifiable only when there is repetitive load as Reuell (2015) has discussed. Also Franklyn-Miller et al. (2009) revealed that the tractus iliotibialis has the largest load on sagittal-plane movement (hip flexion). Fascia latae and its thicker part known as tractus iliotibialis seem to develop under load and therefore it is a great example of how regular DCT is capable of force transmission and how it reacts under load (Fig. 2.13)

Continued

BOX 2.3—**cont'd**

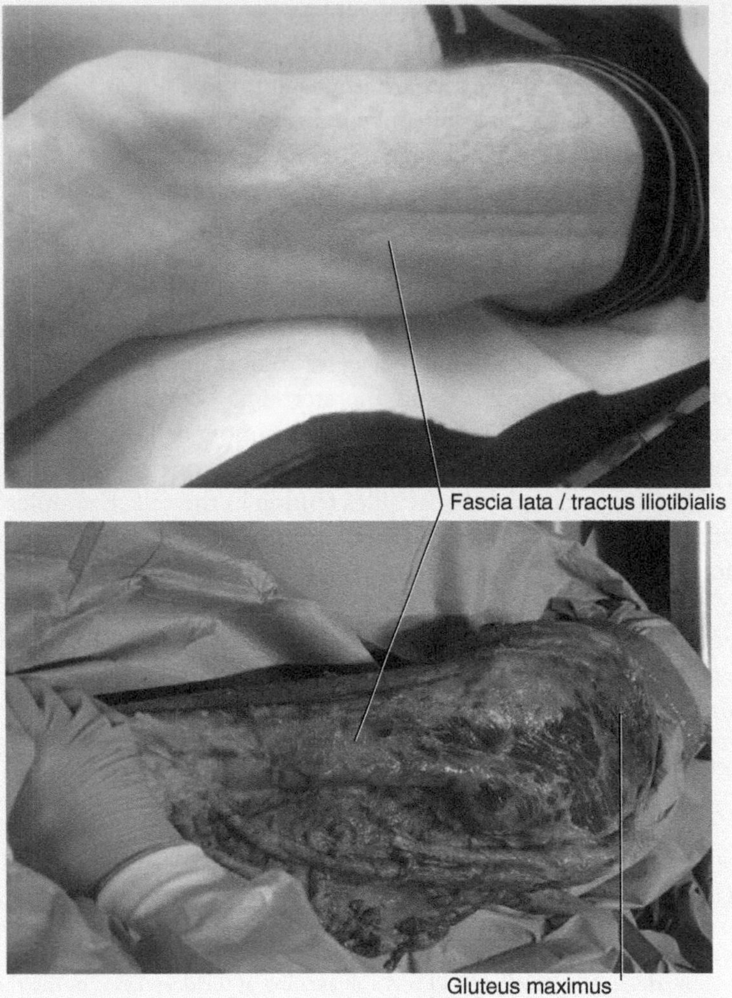

Fig. 2.13 Iliotibial band. Upper image is showing the tensioned fascia latae of a 70-year-old former Olympic rower and strongest man competitor. Lower picture is visualizing fascia latae in a dissection image.

their lives feel and look different from their inactive counterparts. The fascial network is developed in tandem with the muscular frame of the body. These two systems give each person a distinct look and way of moving. We can often recognize acquaintances by the way they move (Magnusson et al., 2010).

Mechanical force transmission (Box 2.4) occurs when muscular tension is applied to deep fascia via the LCT and specifically to stronger connections called

BOX 2.4

The following is a clinical example of fascial force transmission. Kevin, a 54-year-old carpenter, has been active throughout his life. He has been doing heavy lifting for years, but 2 years ago when he was lifting a heavy package, he heard a snapping sound in his right hip. Over the next 6 months he developed increasing amounts of hip and groin pain. He complains of intermittent right hip pain especially upon squatting. He states that the quadriceps area on his right side always feels tight and stretching does not seem to help. Kevin had a history of low back pain 5 years ago but did not feel that it was related to his hip and groin pain.

Examination of hip range of motion was normal except for limited and minimally painful internal rotation. Pelvic external rotation was stiff and limited on the left but not painful. Knee evaluation was negative except for pain during the lunge test at 90° right knee flexion. Knee pain occurred at end range of flexion. Muscle testing of the pelvis and lower extremities was overall 4/5. Treatment was focused on the lateral sequence, to the area of the right iliotibial tract and between the gluteus maximus and medius muscles. The quadratus lumborum muscles were treated bilaterally and balancing of the treatment was performed from the adductor muscle. (This terminology of LA-LU bi, LA-PV rt, LA-GE rt, and ME-GE rt will be more understandable as the book progresses.) After treatment, Kevin was able to squat without pain, internal hip rotation improved, and full knee flexion returned. Muscles tested 5/5. Kevin remarked that he felt stronger and that his movements were smoother. By releasing the tensional dysfunction in the area of his lumbar spine, pelvis, and thigh, Kevin was able to recruit his muscle more precisely and proprioceptive function was apparently restored (Fig. 2.14).

Lieberman et al. (2006) support the idea of the gluteus maximus as a fascial tensor. A major part (80%) of the gluteus maximus is inserted into the fascia latae and its thickened iliotibial tract. The fascia latae covers all the muscles of the thigh like a stocking and it can be visualized as a thick, whitish layer of connective tissue, similar to an aponeurosis (Benninghoff, 1994; Stecco A. et al., 2013a). Coactivation of the pelvis, hip, and thigh region is closely linked to the myofascial system and force transmission occurs via the aponeurotic fascia (fascia latae) (Langevin et al., 2011). The gluteus maximus and medius are covered by epimysial fascia and loose connective

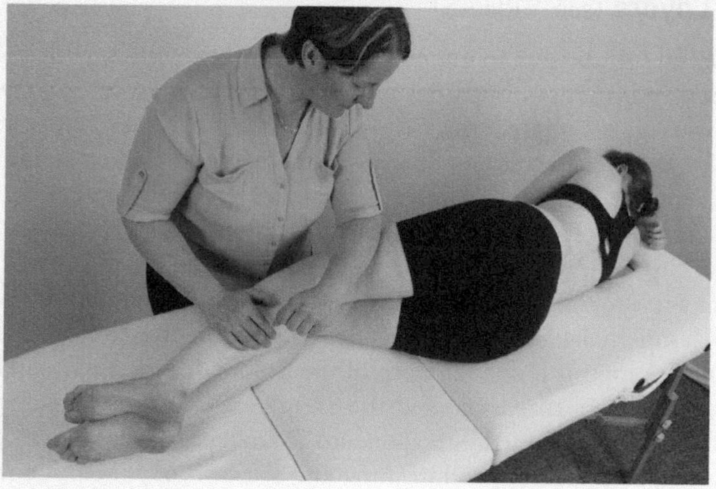

Fig. 2.14 Treatment of the thigh region, side lying, focused towards the LA-GE centre of coordination.

Continued

BOX 2.4—cont'd

tissue that allows the gliding and coordination between these muscles. In Kevin's case, treatment of the lumbar, pelvic, and thigh regions helped to restore hip function. One could hypothesize that the lumbar area may have been the original problem causing compensation of the pelvis, hip, and knee over time. At the least, fascial manipulation offered a logical plan of action, instead of the usual approach that would have concentrated on the site of pain. Antonio Stecco's dissections (2013) have demonstrated these anatomic and functional relationships between the gluteus maximus and fascia latae. In six cadavers, the fascia of the gluteus maximus muscle was continuous with the superficial layer of the posterior lamina of the thoracolumbar fascia and the sacrotuberous ligament and fascia latae below.

fascial expansions (Findley et al., 2012). Thirty-seven percent of muscular attachments are connected to fascial layers and not to bone or tendon (Smeulders et al., 2005). These attachments work like a ship's sail; when it is pulled to one corner it gives the ship direction and force. In the human body, an example of this continuum is from the anterior part of the deltoid muscle toward the biceps brachii muscle. The fascia of the biceps brachii forms the lacertus fibrosus, which covers the part of the forearm flexor attached to the deep fascia. In FM, the centre of fusion (CF) points are located in the retinaculum and myofascial expansion areas. Myofascial expansions are introduced more closely in Chapter 3 of this book. Since the CF points contain a very large amount of proprioceptors that may become densified and inhibited, treating them is essential in order to affect and restore proprioception and force transmission in the myofascial continuum.

Fascial Layers (see Video 5)

Each fascial layer is distinct in important ways from each other, with its own orientation and composition. Superficial fascia, for instance, is loosely packed and irregular, whereas deep fascia is a well-organized fibrous layer. Superficial fascia is formed by interwoven collagen fibres, which are loosely packed and intermixed with abundant elastic fibres. Fat lobules are separated by the membranous layers of superficial fascia (Fig. 2.15). Problems in this layer may appear as swelling, hypersensitivity, or immune response reactions. The depth of superficial fascia varies from a few millimetres to 2 cm under the skin. Mechanoreceptors are present in both superficial and deep fascia. Superficial fascial treatment differs from the deep fascial approach due to depth of the tissues, location of neural components, amount of fascial tension, and the overall effect on the neural system).

Deep fascia can be divided into aponeurotic and epimysial fascia according to its orientation, composition, architecture, and location. Aponeurotic fasciae are formed by two to three layers of parallel bundles of collagen fibres (Fig. 2.16). Each layer is separated from the adjacent one by a thin layer of LCT. Aponeurotic fasciae envelop and connect whole groups of muscles. It covers the muscles of the

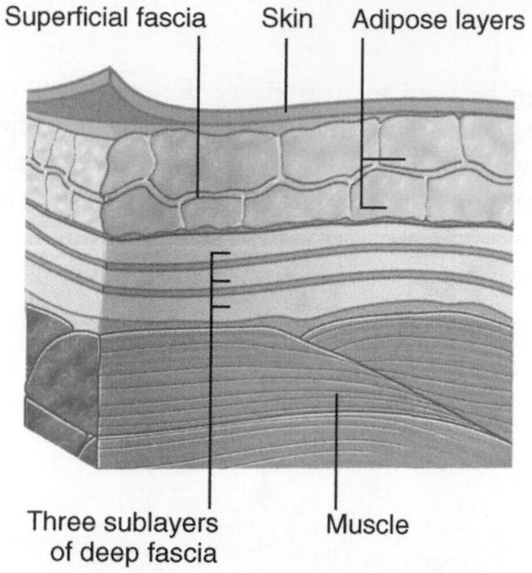

Fig. 2.15 Image of fascial layers.

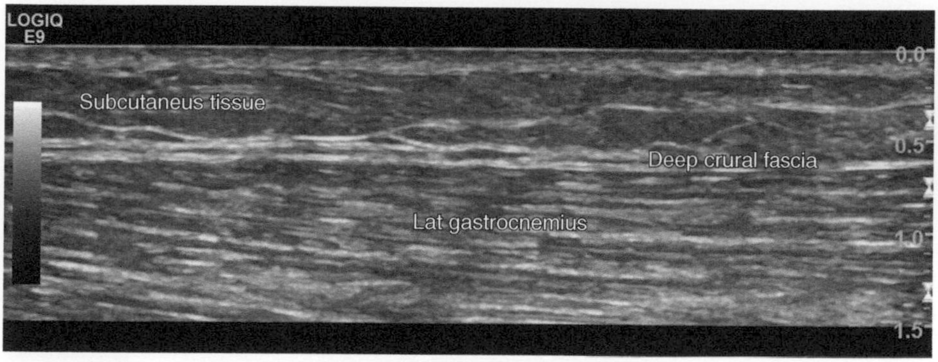

Fig. 2.16 Ultrasound image of the layers from the calf area. *(Courtesy of Jouko Heiskanen, MD.)*

extremities and is located in parts of the trunk, both front and back. Epimysial fasciae cover specifically each muscle, and in the extremities and some parts of the trunk the aponeurotic fascia slides over the epimysial fascia. The epimysial fasciae are locally entwined with individual muscles. Both the aponeurotic fascia and epimysial fascia transmit the force of muscle contraction. Closely associated with the epimysium, which covers the outside of every muscle, is the perimysium that covers the muscle bundles. They contain the spindle cells that are the chief proprioceptors of muscle. Deep fascia will react more easily to deep manipulation using a limited amount of gliding, localized to a small area (Box 2.5). The depth of the deep fascia varies from a few millimetres to couple of centimetres. Overall, the thickness of the deep fascia ranges from 0.5 mm to 1 mm (Stecco et al., 2015).

BOX 2.5

Fascial manipulation can be used to treat either the superficial or deep fascia, but it is primarily focused on the deep fascia and its dysfunctions. Therapists will feel the fascial layers during palpation with the fingers to identify the densified areas. Palpation can thus target treatment appropriately to the correct layer and location. Therapists should keep in mind that the depth of superficial fascia varies from a few millimetres to 2 cm under the skin. The depth of the deep fascia also varies from few millimetres to couple of centimetres (Fig. 2.17).

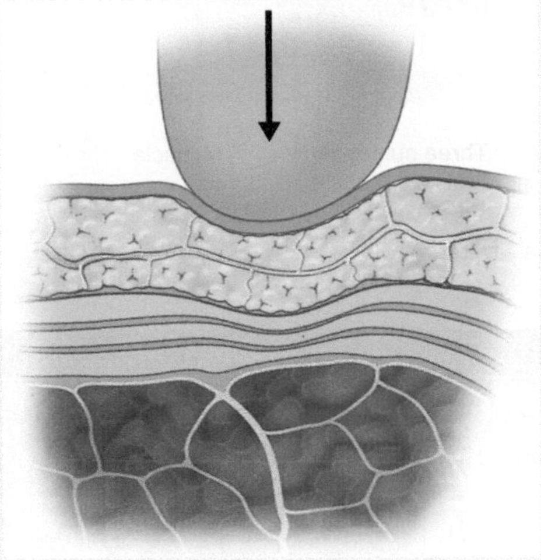

Fig. 2.17 Finger showing pressure through the tissue.

Fascial layers are also present in the internal fascia, and connective tissue both envelops and surrounds organs. Nerves, veins, and glands are surrounded by connective tissue in a variety of forms (Fig. 2.18). The architecture of the epimysium and perimysium of the muscle is similar to the organization of the visceral fascia where the pericardium of the heart and pleura encompass the lungs. According to Luigi Stecco (Stecco and Stecco, 2014) internal fascia can be divided into three categories: visceral, vascular, and glandular. These sheaths can be found in the neck, thoracic, abdominal, and pelvic areas. The CT layers around the larynx and pharynx are defined as the visceral fascia in the neck region, while connective layers around the carotid and jugular arteries are encased by vascular fascia. Glandular fascia encases the thyroid and parathyroid. As explained by Luigi Stecco, these fasciae, as a coordinated network of sheaths, promote organ synchrony. Internal fascia connects and covers the organs. Fascial sheaths coordinate the musculoskeletal system with the organs (Stecco L., 2014) (Fig. 2.19).

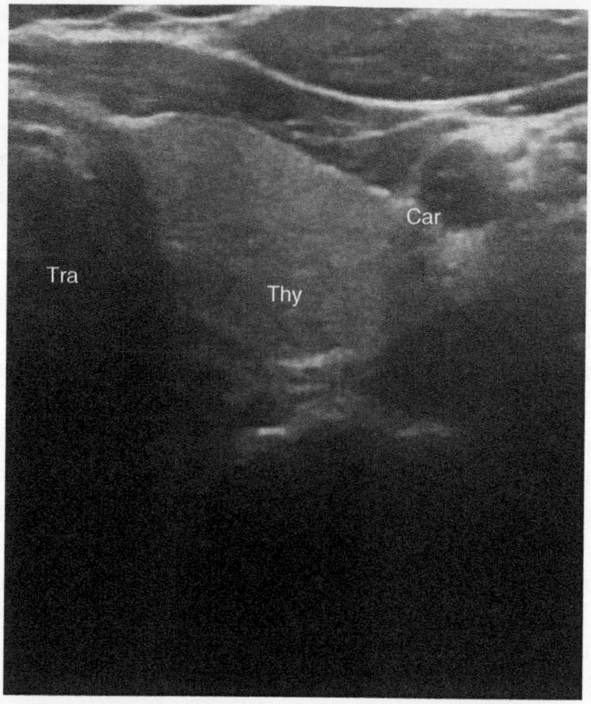

Fig. 2.18 Ultrasound image of the thyroid. Trachea (Tra) is visible in the left side of the thyroid (Thy) and carotid artery (car) in the right side. *(Image courtesy of Jouko Heiskanen, MD.)*

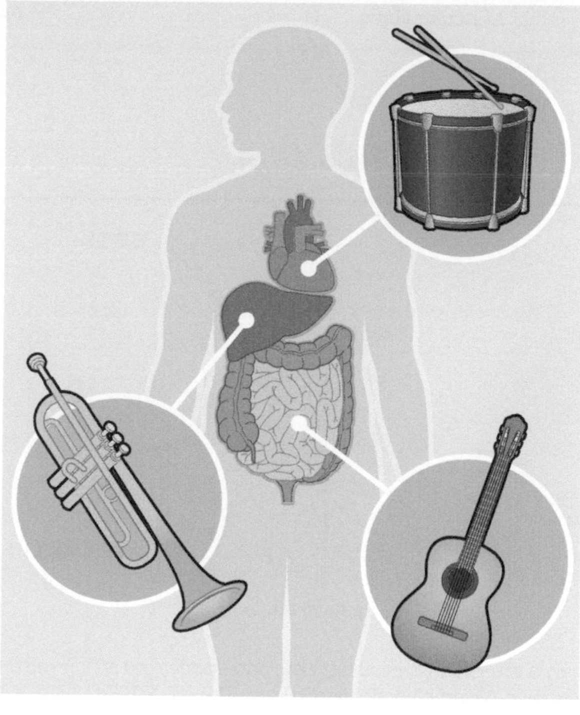

Fig. 2.19 Internal organs and the fascial connections can be visualized as instruments in orchestra. They should be in synchrony and harmony to create beautiful concerto.

HYALURONAN

It is possible to find HA (Fig. 2.20) everywhere in the human body. It exists in all CT from the periosteum to the skin. For instance, HA is used on the skin by the beauty industry to make the skin appear younger, more lubricated, and more elastic. In the musculoskeletal system, HA is ubiquitous, especially between the layers of the aponeurotic fascia, between the deep fascia and muscles, in the LCT surrounding muscle bundles, and within the intramuscular fascial layers, that is, the epimysium, perimysium, and endomysium (Fig. 2.21).

HA-secreting cells termed fasciacytes have also been identified not only in the deep fascia but also in the retinaculum. One of the many functions of HA is to act as a lubricant (protecting normal tissue viscosity) allowing all of the above fascial layers to glide upon one another. Another HA function is to protect muscles. HA is found throughout the extracellular matrix. When tissue is injured, HA stimulates satellite muscle cell proliferation, which is necessary for muscle tissue healing. After an injury (eg, hamstring strain), the healing process always begins with inflammation. In a simple model, inflammation works like construction workers in a new building. If you want to create a sturdy building, you have to first create a new base for the building and establish a strong foundation. Inflammation promotes this process and one role of HA is to open the tissue spaces through which cells can travel. Inflammation is a worker and HA is a control unit allowing

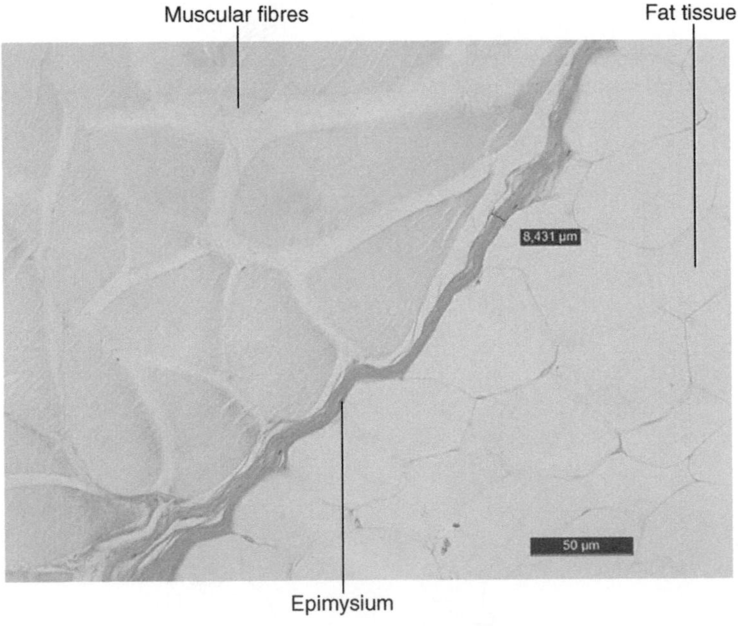

Fig. 2.20 Hyaluronan is present in the muscle cells and epimysium is rich with HA. This is visible in the microscopic view with Alcian blue staining. *(From Stecco, 2013.)*

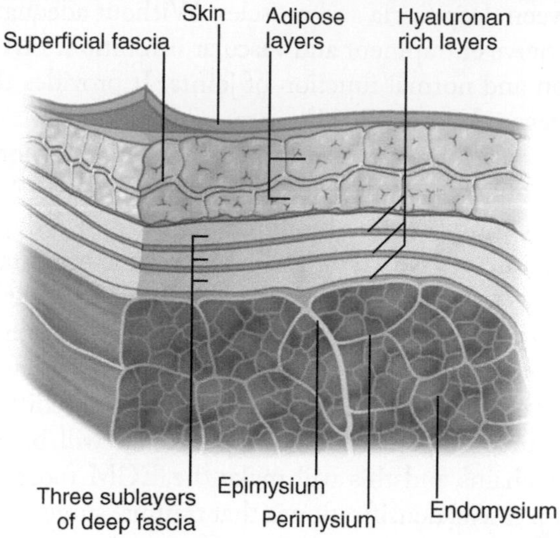

Fig. 2.21 Deep fascial layers are rich with HA.

freight travelling to the construction site. HA is prominent not only in the injury recovery process, but also during embryogenesis in tissues undergoing rapid growth and during the repair and regeneration processes. HA is abundant during the earliest stages of wound healing, where it stimulates satellite cell proliferation.

A definite amount of water/fluid is crucial for cellular function, especially to allow cells to tolerate mechanical stress, such as tension via pulling and increased intracellular pressure created by tension. Water content also affects the state of the ground substance (ie, the gel-to-sol phenomenon). Low water content means a more solid state that increases the friction between the collagen fibres. This, in turn, limits their capacity to be mobile. Changes in the GAGs, including their main constituent HA (Box 2.6), contribute to pain, inflammation, and loss of function (Stecco C., 2015a).

HA also serves an important function in both perivascular and perineural areas. In the perivascular areas, especially around veins, and in the perineural areas around nerves, normal properties of HA are necessary to allow adequate gliding of fascia and LCT on these structures. This relationship is similar to the

BOX 2.6

Hyaluronan (HA) is one of the key elements in fascial manipulation (FM). Alteration of the extracellular matrix and its relation to fascia is considered to be associated with the cause of myofascial pain (Stecco et al., 2011). The effect of FM on HA using deep compression and friction over particular locations within the fascia is probably one of the main reasons for the success of this method.

relationship between deep fascia and muscles. Without adequate gliding there is the potential for nerve entrapment and vascular inhibition. HA is also important for the lubrication and normal function of joints. It provides the lubrication for synovial fluid (Stecco A. et al., 2011).

Changes in viscoelasticity can lead to a loss of range of motion, muscle stiffness, pain, and eventually inflammation. Like all cells, GAG cells have a specific turnover time. HA turnover time is approximately 2 to 4 days while the other GAGs have a lifetime of 7 to 10 days. Therefore it is important for patients to keep active. Inactivity or static activities like sitting in front of the computer for hours and hours every day are risk factors for a change in the quantity and quality of the ground substance (Stecco, 2015). FM targets its treatment to restore the viscoelastic properties of the tissues and to modify the alterations in the ground substance rich with HA. Deep friction will break the cross-links between the HA chains and this will make the ECM more fluid and flexible. A prime reason for fascial densification is that trauma, surgery, overuse, or misuse could cause fragmentation of the HA molecules that promote inflammation and an increase in viscosity. Increased viscosity can result in stiffness, pain, and loss of motion due to the viscous effect on the free nerve endings and mechanoreceptors that are necessary for painless muscle function. The HA chains could become entangled, increase in concentration and viscosity, and prevent normal gliding between fascia and muscles. HA entanglement can be normalized by increased temperature (40 °C) and freeing of fibres. Unfortunately, many soft tissue methods whose main effect is to mainly increase temperature may only provide short-term relief. It is necessary to provide enough compression and friction to alter the gliding properties of fascial layers in relation to each other. This has been demonstrated through ultrasonographic imaging (Fig. 2.22) (Luomala et al., 2014; Stecco A. et al., 2013b).

Retinacula

As previously mentioned, the treatment of retinacula is considered extremely important in FM. Retinacula are the site of CF and contain the most mechanoreceptors of the fascia. The term retinaculum is derived from the Latin *retinere*, to restrain, or *rete*, a net (Box 2.7). Retinacula have been described as structures that restrain an organ or tissue in place or as a network of collagen fibre bundles that form a cross pattern. They are connective tissue bundles located near joints, such as the knee, ankle, elbow, and wrist. Retinacula resemble ligaments, but their composition and function differ. Composed of regular connective tissue, ligaments bind two bones together acting as a supporting structure for joints. Retinacula are actually reinforcements of the deep fascia attaching to joint capsules, bones, muscles, and tendons and can also fuse with the superficial fascia (Fig. 2.23).

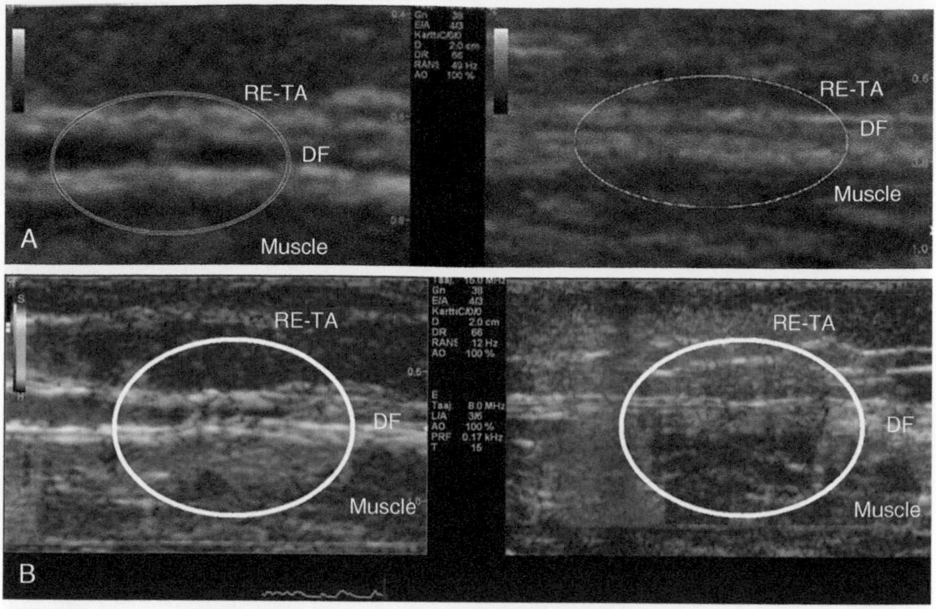

FIG. 2.22 Densified CC, in the ultrasonography image. (A) Ultrasonography image of RE-TA point. RE-TA is centre of coordination, which is located over the fascia of lateral gastrocnemius muscle. (B) Elastography image of RE-TA point. Left side image shows situation before treatment and right side after the FM treatment. Blue color in elastography is indicating stiff tissue (viscoelastic properties are altered), green color shows some stiffness in the tissue and red color marks soft and elastic tissue. *(From Luomala, 2014.)*

BOX 2.7

Ligament and retinaculum are not similar structures: Ligament (Latin *ligamentum* = bond) bonds two bones together and has a resistant structure, with fibres that are arranged along a rather uniform line of traction. Retinaculum (Latin *rete* = net) is a network or grid of collagen fibres arranged according to multiple lines of traction.

Retinacula consist of collagen fibres arranged in layers, with each layer oriented in a different direction (similar to aponeurotic fascial layers). Their network of fibres cross over each other and at the same time slide independently from one another. Ensuring the sliding of retinacula layers is extremely important for continued joint proprioception and pain reduction. They also continue in a helicoidal pattern, along the various fascial CF sequences, forming a spiral. These spiral sequences are treated in FM and will be discussed later in the book, see Chapter 4 (Stecco C., 2015a).

From a classic point of view, retinacula are described as a passive type of tissue. Probably the most commonly known retinacula are in the wrist and ankle areas, where they stabilize the muscles and tendons. Since the time of Vesalius (1543), retinacula have been designated as pulley systems or more lately as a load-shear

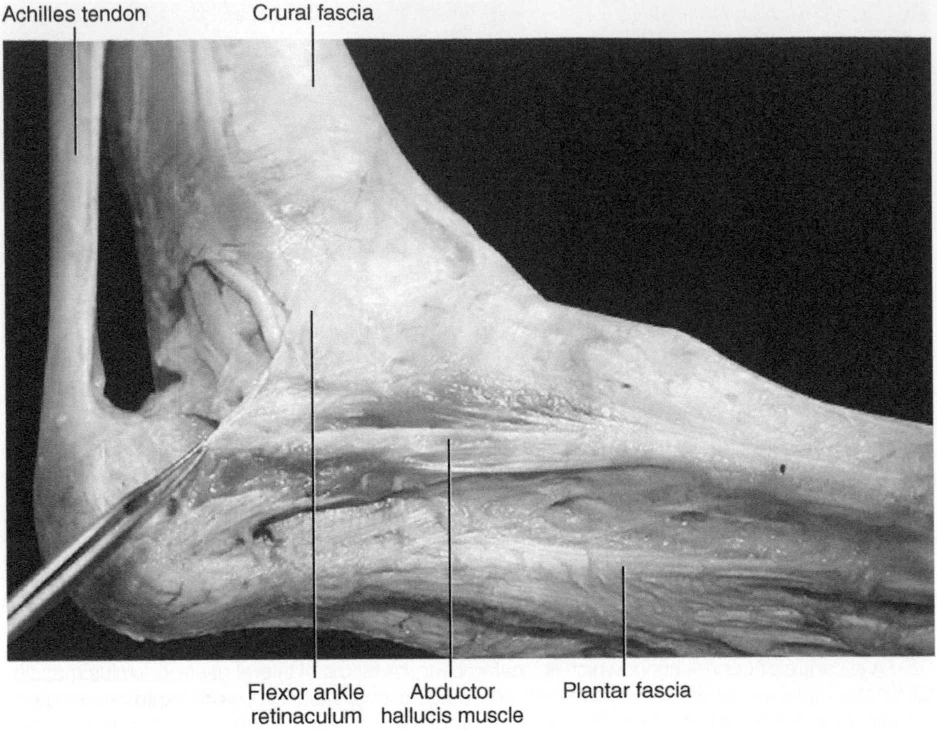

Fig. 2.23 Dissection image of ankle retinaculum shows fascial connections and orientation of retinacula areas. *(From Stecco, 2013.)*

system (Powers et al., 2006). As a pulley system, retinacula hold tendons in their position and simultaneously give tendons the ability to work more powerfully. A reinvestigation of anatomy demonstrates that retinacula are not principally a passive stabilizing or pulley system for tendons and muscles. Rather, retinacula are three-layered structures containing layers of collagen fibres, which are able to glide independently from one another within the ECM. If retinacula were just a tendon holder, why do they have such complex structures? A monolayered structure, as in ligaments, would be sufficient for a pulley system.

Complexity of retinacular architecture reveals a functionally complex action. Another interesting fact about retinacular anatomy is its innervation. Retinacula are the most highly innervated fascial tissue, rich in free nerve endings and Ruffini and Pacinian corpuscles. Obviously they are much more than a passive stabilizer. Retinacula should be seen as specialized proprioceptive organs that perceive joint movement. Retinacula have connections to muscle and bone, which makes them able to sense both bone movement and muscular contraction. Retinacula have a connective tissue system allowing them to have a stabilizing role, but with its complex multilayered structure and rich innervation it supports the idea of also acting as a proprioceptive organ rather than just a passive stabilizing system (Stecco et al., 2010).

A basic three-layered histological composition of the extensor retinacula is repeated in anatomic pulleys throughout the body (Klein et al., 1999). But there are elements that support the hypothesis of other functions for the retinacula:

1. The superior retinaculum of the extensor muscles of the foot is situated at the inferior third of the leg where tendons do not require retinacular support as they might under the inferior retinaculum.
2. If the only role of the inferior retinaculum of the foot were that of a restraint, then all of its fibres would be inserted onto bone, instead of which many of its fibres continue with the posterior fascia (Box 2.8).
3. Around the knee, the patellar retinaculum and the popliteal retinaculum do not maintain any tendons close to the bone.
4. In the wrist, the transverse carpal ligament restrains the flexor tendons while the flexor retinaculum is effectively independent and slides over the ligament.

Retinacula are present in all articulations. They are connected to tendons and are more or less visible depending on the load to which they have been subjected to over time.

BOX 2.8

The retinacula of the ankle are structures that researchers have attempted to define in various ways. Stecco (2010) studied 27 dissected ankles. In this study, magnetic resonance imaging was performed *in vivo* in seven healthy subjects, 17 subjects with sprained ankles, and three with an amputated limb. This study demonstrated that the retinacula of the ankle are reinforcements of the deep fascia. This fact may explain why so many define this structure in different ways. The retinaculum of the ankle is now considered more of a dynamic than static structure. Stress makes it stronger and thicker while inactivity makes the retinaculum thinner. Fibre orientation and innervation findings support this. Retinacula contain, based on their size, the largest amount of mechanical receptors in the body. Thus, after an ankle sprain it is crucial that function be restored to this important structure. In addition, examination should ascertain what other structures might be involved via the leg (crural fascia) extending toward the limbs and pelvis (fascia latae). The mechanism of the trauma will guide the therapist to the sequence of the injury—how to examine it and how to restore both proprioception and movement to the impaired area. Based on fascial manipulation (FM) studies, retinacula are not static structures for joint stabilization, like ligaments, but act as a specialized fascial reinforcement for local spatial proprioception of joints.

The following is a typical case responding to FM. Catherine, age 55 years, is a physiotherapist who owns her own company. Besides work, she is very active, including volleyball and jogging. Her chief complaint is that her left leg feels weak, with a feeling of "giving way, " especially when jumping during volleyball. Her history includes a 10-year-old ligamentous tear on the left lateral side of her ankle that occurred during a volleyball game. It took a year of rehabilitation before she was able to play again. During the succeeding years she was not aware of ankle pain, but intermittently over the years she has complained of knee and leg pain in the

Continued

BOX 2.8—cont'd

left lower limb. Movement and palpation verification revealed a dysfunctional spiral originating in her left foot. Treatment extended from the foot to the knee and pelvis. After a few treatments by FM her leg felt balanced and she no longer complained of pain. This case is a typical example of how a previous injury becomes responsible for a present complaint. Feelings of physical awkwardness, joint instability, and uncontrolled movements are common complaints of the majority of the population. One of the great contributions of FM is its ability to evaluate and treat the fascial kinetic chain (Fig. 2.24).

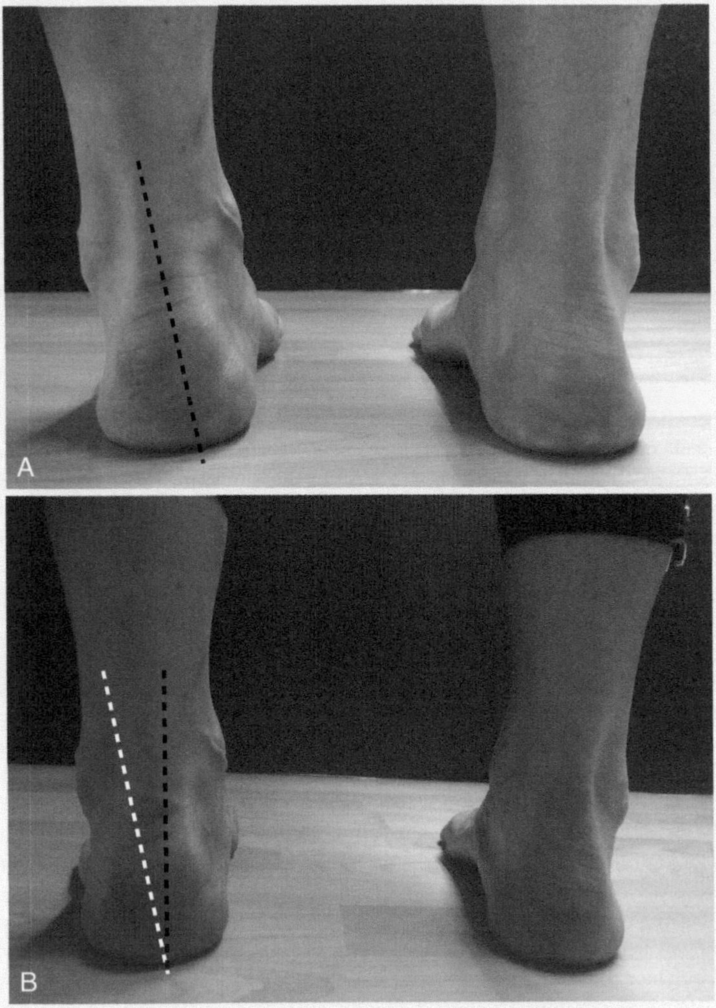

Fig. 2.24 (A) Before FM treatment, black line indicates alignment of calcaneus. (B) After treatment, white line indicates original alignment and black line indicates results of the FM treatment.

A Muscle—the Center of the Myofascial Force Transmission

Force is created by muscular tissue *(myo)*. At the cellular level, a muscle cell is the smallest fascia-related structure. It is also known as muscle fibre. It is fascia-related because each muscle cell is enveloped by a membrane called the endomysium that strongly adheres to the surrounding tissues. Muscle cells form bundles of muscle cells called fasciculi (fascicles, muscle bundles), which in turn are covered by a membrane called the perimysium. The individual fibres are surrounded by endomysium. The fascia surrounding the whole muscle is called the epimysium. DCT exists especially in perimysium and epimysium. The perimysium is the densest CT (Drake et al., 2015) (Fig. 2.25).

Muscle cells are composed of smaller parts known as myofibrils. Myofibrils contain sarcomeres, which are formed by actin, myosin, and titin filaments. These structures can only be identified under a microscope. The interaction of these myofibrillar proteins allows muscles to contract. Contraction occurs when the muscle fibre receives a stimulus (the action potential) from the nervous system. This electrical stimulus causes Ca^{2+} to be released from the sarcoplasmic reticulum. Calcium then binds the actin and myosin heads together. As long as Ca^{2+} and adenosine triphosphate are present, the myosin heads will attach to the actin molecules, pull the actin, release, and reattach (Davies, 1963).

The electrical stimulus to the muscle cell is transferred via a motor neuron. Motor neurons come in two categories, upper and lower motor neurons. The upper motor neurons originate from the motor cortex and terminate in the spinal cord. Lower motor neurons originate from the spinal cord, anterior grey column, anterior nerve roots, or cranial nerve nuclei of the brainstem. The lower motor neurons (alpha motor neuron) terminate in the motor end plates within the endomysium of a muscle cell/fibre. An individual motor neuron and all the muscle fibres it innervates is called a motor unit. The average amount of the muscle cells innervated by one motor unit is approximately 100 to 200. Innervation of the muscle cells varies. Muscles used for fine movements have motor neurons that will innervate only a small number of muscle fibres. For instance, the m. orbicularis oculi may consist of only five muscle cells per motor neuron; whereas the m. gluteus maximus may contain as many as 2000 muscle cells for each motor neuron. In other words, muscles with a large number of muscle cells in one motor unit are used for posture or coarse movements. The motor unit is the smallest functional unit (Hamill and Knutzen, 2009; Knierim, 1997) (Box 2.9, Fig. 2.26). The contractile properties of a motor unit are based on the structural characteristics of its muscle fibres. The motor fibres are divided into three subgroups: slow twitch oxidative, fast twitch oxidative, and fast twitch glycolytic. When an electrical stimulus arrives at the motor end plates, it will activate all the muscle fibres with similar biochemical and histologic properties of the particular motor unit (Scott et al., 2001).

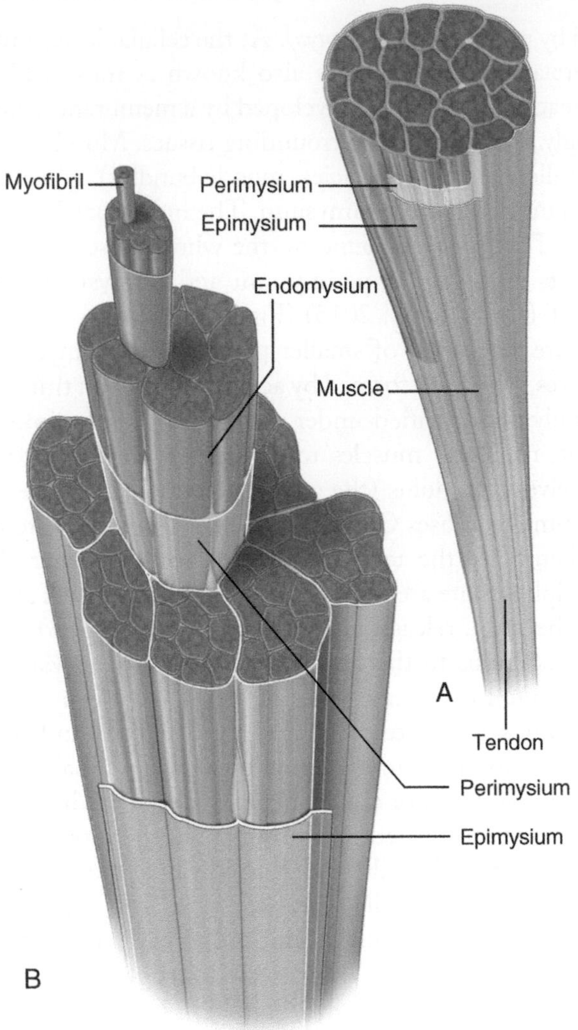

Fig. 2.25 Muscle's fascial system—continuum of the fascial components.

Muscle Spindle

The chief proprioceptor in the muscle system is the muscle spindle cell whose capsule is in the perimysium extending to the epimysium. When a muscle contracts there are two motor nerves from the central nervous system (CNS) that affect muscles: the alpha motor neuron, which is responsible for the muscle contraction (makes up the motor unit), and the gamma motor neuron. The main

BOX 2.9 From the Motor Unit to the Myofascial Unit

The motor unit is one of the basic terms when talking about neuromuscular function. Function of the motor unit relates to function of the muscle spindles. In fascial manipulation, all motor units that control a specific movement direction are called myofascial units (see Chapter 4).

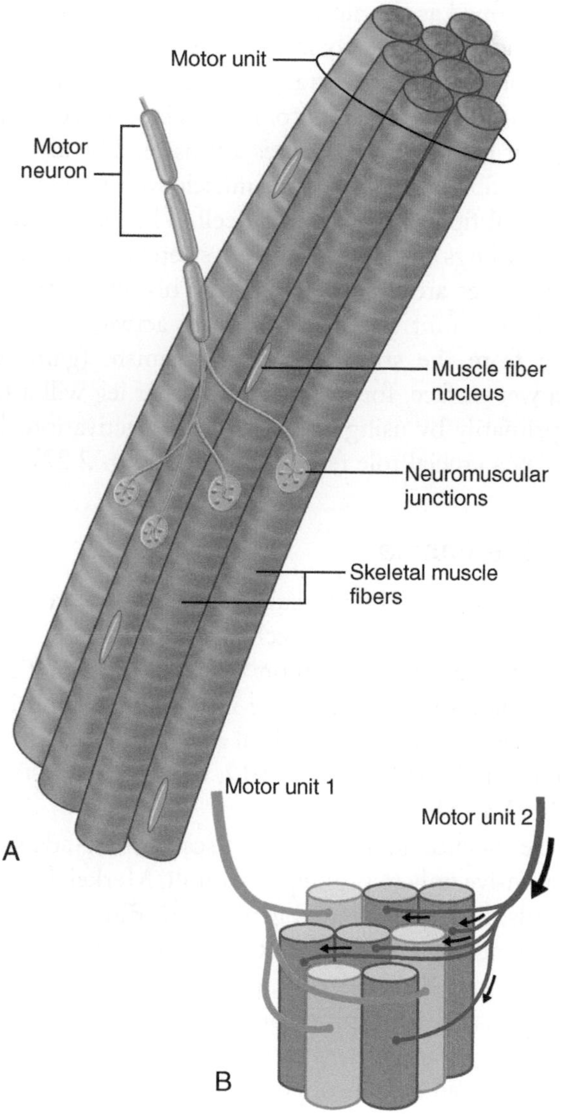

Fig. 2.26 Muscle cell to muscle and motor unit.

responsibility of the gamma motor nerve is to regulate the spindle cell. The importance of the spindle cell is emphasized by the fact that the gamma nerve represents 31% of the motor input from the CNS to the muscle. The information transmitted to the CNS by the muscle spindle cell during muscle contraction and even when the muscle is in a passive state is the state of the muscle contraction, that is, its tone, movement, loss of elasticity, absolute muscle length, position of the muscle in space, and rate of change of muscle length. One of the great effects of FM is to normalize the function of the spindle cell.

A motor unit is defined as the alpha motor neuron and the extrafusal fibres it supplies. Muscle spindle cells, mostly in the belly of the muscle, consist of intrafusal fibres with a noncontractile central region that contains the sensory nerves that report to the CNS. The gamma motor neuron is another motor neuron along with the alpha motor neuron that activates a muscle. The alpha motor neurons activate the extrafusal fibres that supply the muscle with power, while the gamma regulates the intrafusal fibres of the spindle cell. The gamma does this by contracting the polar endings of the cell, which stretches the noncontractile area where the sensory nerves are then stimulated. This allows the maintenance of spindle tautness. Motor unit contraction can be activated via efferent gamma impulses resulting from the stretch reflex mechanism (gamma loop). When one leg slips on a wet surface, for instance, the other leg will attempt to restore upright posture primarily by using alpha-gamma coactivation. In this case the muscle spindles play a crucial role (see Chapter 3) (Fig. 2.27).

Innervation of the Fascia

The main sensory receptors in the musculoskeletal system are the proprioceptors (mechanoreceptors). They transfer mechanical distortion that sends nerve impulses to the CNS. Mechanoreceptors work as part of the fascial system (Box 2.10). Many studies demonstrate the importance of mechanoreceptors in the fascial layers and especially the superficial and middle layers of the deep fascia that are highly innervated (Schleip et al., 2012; Stecco et al., 2007; Stilwell, 1957; Tezars et al., 2011; Van Der Wal, 2009).

Ruffini corpuscles or endings and Merkel discs are slow-adapting touch receptors. They are responsive only to prolonged stimuli. Merkel discs are abundant in the fingertips, hands, lips, and external genitals. Ruffini endings lie deep in the dermis, ligaments, tendons, and fasciae. Ruffini corpuscles are most sensitive to stretch resulting from muscle movement, particularly movement in the limbs or digits. Meissner corpuscles are rapid-adapting touch receptors that react at the onset of a stimulus. They are located in hairless skin. Pacinian corpuscles react to pressure against a broad area as opposed to a localized touch area. They are rapidly adapting receptors and are located in the dermis and subcutaneous tissue, muscles, tendons, and joints. Ruffini and Pacinian corpuscles are both present in fascia and retinacula (Stecco and Stecco, 2012).

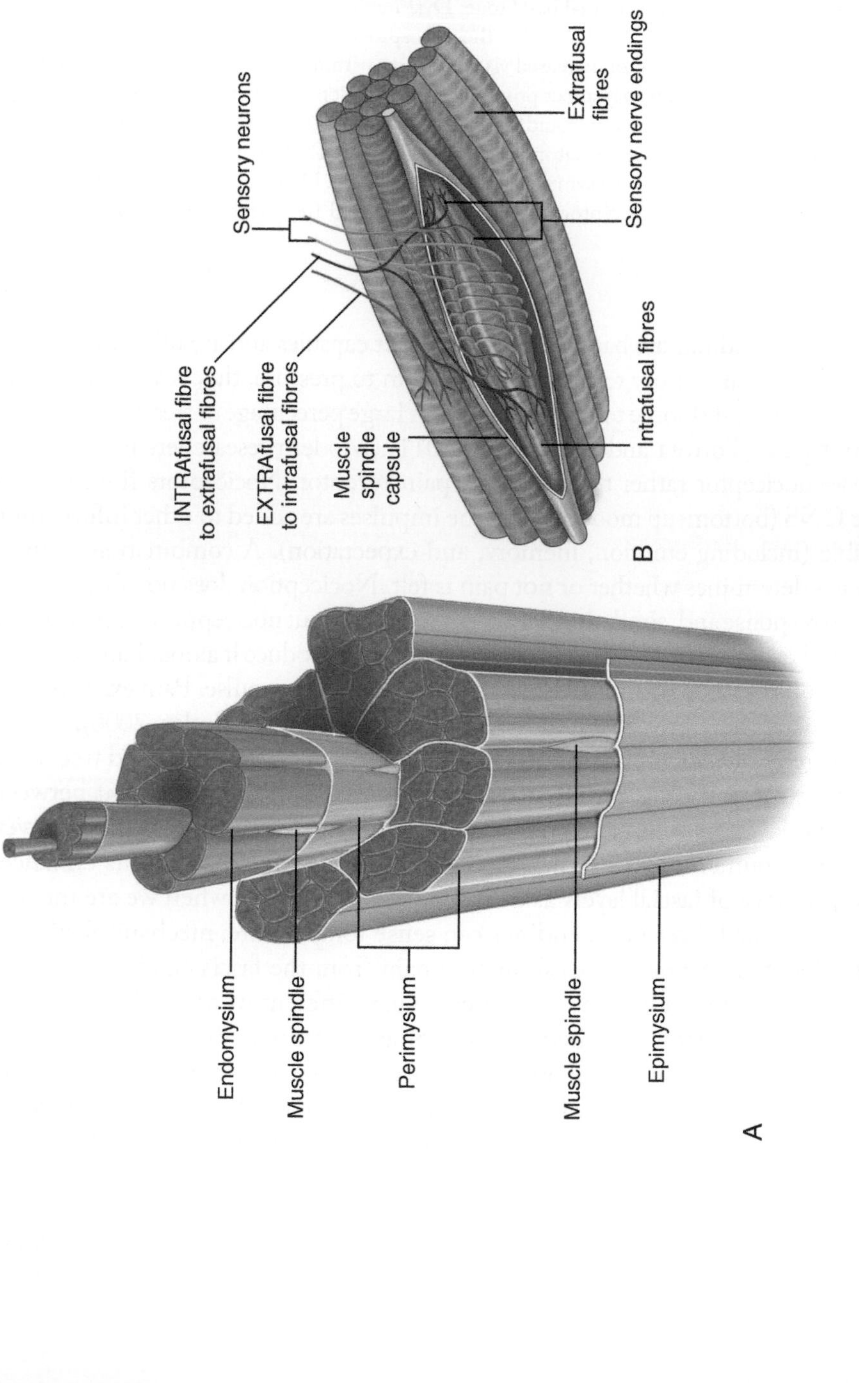

Fig. 2.27 (A) Muscle spindle as a part of myofascial system, located between the perimysium and epimysium. (B) Muscle spindle covered with fascia.

BOX 2.10

We have many receptors in the myofascial system such as Ruffini, Pacinian, and free nerve endings. Fascial manipulation (FM) highlights the treatment of muscle spindles and Golgi tendon organs (GTOs). Correct function of these receptors is dependent on adequate fascial tension or what is known as normal basal tone. Dysfunction of fascial tension alters the action of these receptors. FM strives to normalize these receptors, which become dysfunctional (densified) due to localized areas of increased viscoelasticity within and surrounding the receptors. Altered mechanoreceptors may affect proprioceptive function and change the central nervous system's response. This alteration could affect muscle tone by way of the motor units involved. Responses may also occur via the autonomic nervous system. Ruffini nerve endings have a particularly close connection to the sympathetic nervous system. Hypothalamic and fluid dynamics also stimulate mechanoreceptors, especially Ruffini and free nerve endings (Schleip and Müller, 2012).

Free nerve endings are bare dendrites without capsules and are ubiquitous in the body. They act as sensory receptors. In addition to pressure, they react to temperature, tickle, itch, and some touch sensations. A large percentage of free nerve endings transmit pain (Tortora and Derrickson, 2011). Modern researchers use the term work-as-nociceptor rather than work-as-pain receptor. Nociceptors fire impulses to the CNS (bottom-up model) where the impulses are added to other information available (including emotion, memory, and expectation). A combination of these elements determines whether or not pain is felt. Nociception does not always result in a pain response and, similarly, there can be pain without nociception. Pain is always an individual experience and no human receptor can produce it alone. Pain response depends on the value that the CNS assigns to a received impulse. Pain exists only in the brain and therefore the top–down model is more useful (Butler, 2000).

Collagen fibres surround and attach to the capsules of corpuscles and free nerve endings. Ruffini, Pacini corpuscles, and free nerve endings are present between the fascial layers as well. The amount of free nerve endings may be up to seven times more numerous than other mechanoreceptors (Fig. 2.28). This enhances the importance of fascial layers as a sensory system, sensing when we are moving or being touched. Free nerve endings can sense temperature, mechanical stimuli, and nociception. Some studies show that pain from the fascia can be even more aggravating than pain from muscles. People use different words to describe pain. Fascial pain is usually described as a stabbing, irritating, stinging, or a beating sensation. Muscle pain on the other hand is described as a more dull and aching type of pain (Schilder et al., 2014). This indicates that different anatomic locations can produce different sensory feedback. A skilful therapist can make use of this during a diagnostic examination.

The fascial architecture of the nerve and muscle has similarities. The nerve trunk is surrounded by epineurium and the neuron is enveloped by endoneurium. The muscle is surrounded by epimysium, the fascicles by perineurium, and the

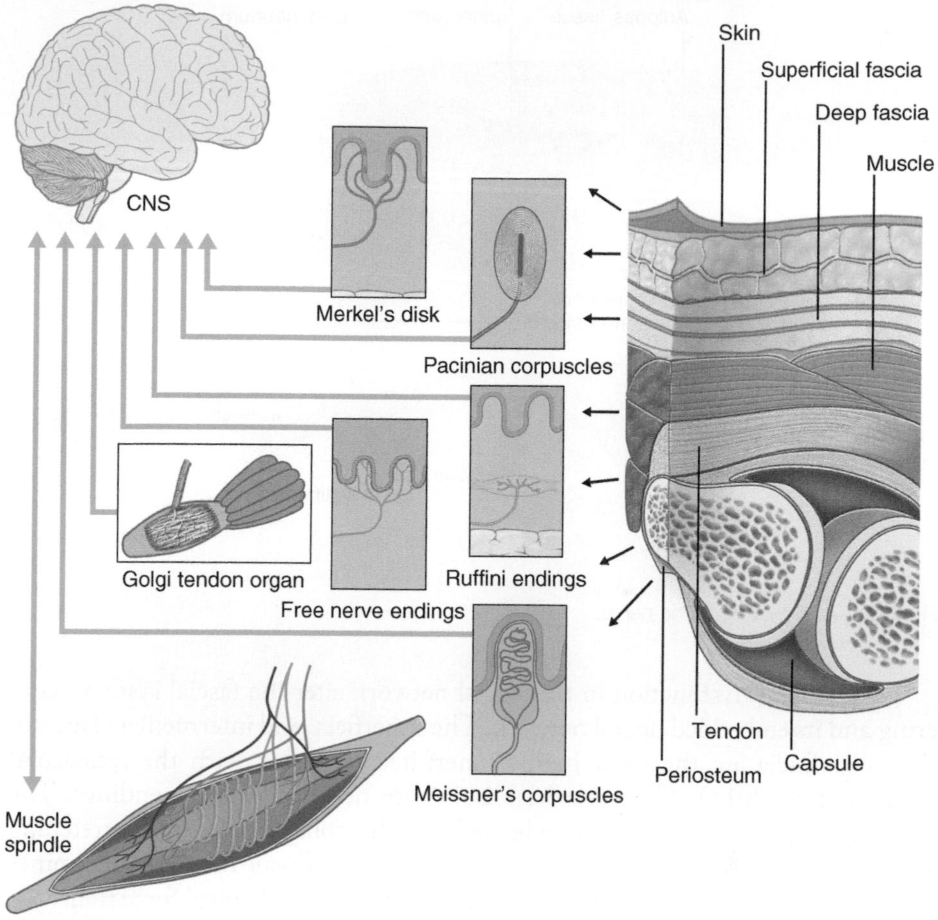

Fig. 2.28 Mechanoreceptors.

fibres by endomysium (Fig. 2.29). Fascial continuity is present from the meninges of the brain and spinal cord to the peripheral nerves. There are three types of peripheral nerves: sensory neurons, 43%; motor neurons, 17%; and sympathetic neurons, 40% (Shepherd and Abboud, 1977). In one nerve trunk (ie, sciatic nerve) both efferent and afferent axons are present, so the traffic of the impulses is two ways. Each individual nerve cell, however, conducts impulses in one direction only. As a rule, nerves have more sensory fibres than motor ones, so there is more traffic toward the brain than away from it. A nerve may be compared to London's underground network, while CNS function would be all of Europe's undergrounds together. In this analogy, one tunnel of the underground system is afferent or efferent so that traffic is one way only. The underground moves people from place to place; similarly, the nervous system sends and receives messages throughout the body.

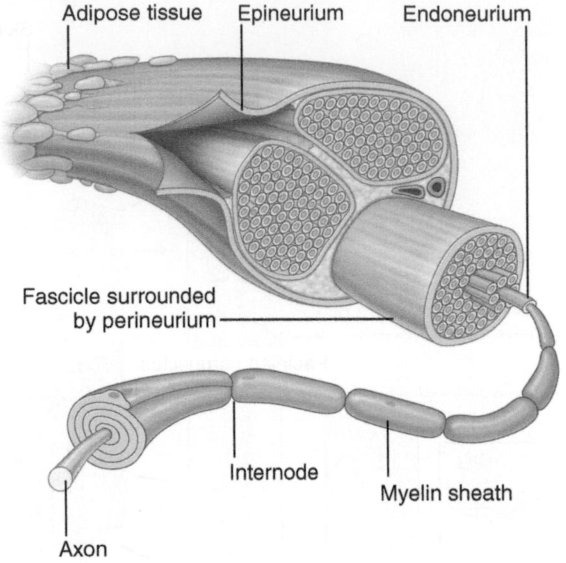

Fig. 2.29 Architecture of the nerve.

Tension and dysfunction in the fascial network alter the fascial system's covering and its embedded neural network. The superficial and intermediate layers of the deep fascia are the most highly innervated (together with the retinacula) (Tezars et al., 2011). The superficial tissues are rich in free nerve endings. The nerve endings are aligned perpendicularly to the collagen fibres, so stretching the muscle and fascia easily stimulates these receptors. Tissue function determines the amount of receptors in different parts of the body. Mechanical force transmission by way of the proprioceptive system is necessary in different parts of our body and determines the number of mechanoreceptors that will be available and also the myofascial kinetic chain. Also viscoelastic changes in the tissues may alter the activation of the mechanoreceptors (Stecco C., 2015a).

Functionality of the Connective Tissue (see Video 6)

The anatomy of connective tissue is interlinked with its function. Modern medicine tends to look at the body as a collection of distinct parts and systems. While this point of view is informative, it misses information on whole system functionality. Concepts such as meridians and muscle chains link the body in a more complex and functional way (Langevin, 2006). FM combines segments and systems as functional elements of the whole body. Problems in our body do not leap from area to area but rather travel along the body's communication and functional network (Box 2.11).

BOX 2.11

An example of this functional fascial network is pain or stiffness in the shoulder area. When examining the shoulder or for that matter any joint, it is necessary to examine not only the joint but all of the surrounding tissues such as the muscles, ligaments, and fascia. One test to determine the complete range of shoulder motion is humeroscapular rhythm. For example, if the scapula is stabilized and prevented from moving, the humerus will move from 90° to 105° before the scapula moves. For further abduction and for all shoulder joint motion, the whole upper extremity myofascial system must function in a coordinated manner. In most trauma or overuse of the shoulder, in order to diminish pain, compensations occur. The scapula's range of motion is increased, some muscles may become overactive or underactive and proprioception will be altered. The patient is now clearly uncoordinated. The myofascial system now requires more energy, endurance, and strength causing adjoining areas such as the neck, scapula, elbow, or wrist to become overactive. These dysfunctions are visible when testing movement verification before palpation and fascial manipulation (FM) treatment (Fig. 2.30).

A 51-year-old shopkeeper had pain, stiffness, and loss of range of motion in her left shoulder joint area. Flexion of the shoulder joint was 145°, abduction 110°, and with the hand-behind-back-test she was unable to reach her gluteal area (indicating a loss of shoulder internal rotation and extension). Her pain slowly increased during a 5- to 6-month period, to the level of 7/10 (VAS). She also complained of night pain affecting her sleep. There was also pain in her left forearm and stiffness in her left wrist. Eventually the stiffness spread bilaterally to her neck with occasional occipital headaches. About 1 year ago she fell down and broke her forearm (fracture of the left radius). It was immobilized for 1 month. It was hypothesized that her

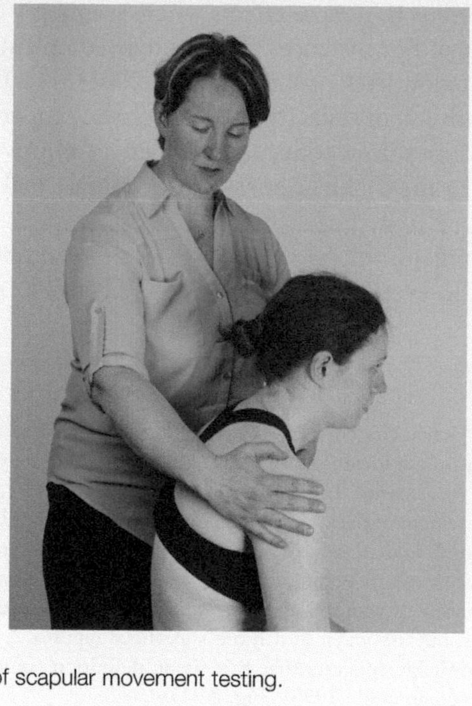

Fig. 2.30 Example of scapular movement testing.

Continued

BOX 2.11—cont'd

past injury (fracture of the radius and prolonged immobilization) may have resulted in compensatory shoulder and neck pain. FM palpatory verification of the myofascial sequences revealed painful densifications along the anterior and lateral parts of her forearm and in the neck area. The most intense painful and densified points (centres of coordination, centres of fusion) were located in the anterior distal region over the forearm and wrist retinaculum. Immediately after the FM treatment of the lower forearm and wrist, her shoulder movements significantly increased with diminished pain. After 3 visits that included neck treatment, her headache was gone and shoulder joint mobility was restored. Interestingly, her shoulder pain was compensatory and did not require treatment.

Fascia also participates in mechanotransduction (mechanisms by which cells convert mechanical stimulus into electrochemical activity). Cells perceive and interpret tension and mechanical forces through the fascia. Enduring or long-term mechanical forces remodel connective tissue. It is hypothesized that cells have a "memory." Sensory deprivation has been studied in humans and apes. Primates seem to need touching. Could memories and feelings be stored in the myofascial system as well? Our connective tissue can react bioelectrically, by cell-to-cell communication or with tissue plasticity responses. This interaction between tissues may play a significant role in understanding pathological changes in our body and also may lead us to remote effects where seemingly unrelated areas and systems react to trauma. For instance, patients may complain of stomach symptoms that are related to low back pain (Langevin, 2006). Treatment and touching can affect both our movement capacity and viscoelastic properties between fascial layers (Box 2.12). FM uses these concepts and thereby improves mechanical force transmission by freeing the dysfunctional areas (Luomala et al., 2014; Siddhartha et al., 2009).

Our body development results in precise layers of embedded fascia. This process is present in every stage of our life. Tension continually creates

BOX 2.12

Old Chinese exercises like tai chi, chi kung (qi kong), lian kong or Indian traditions of yoga-exercise may be healthy for our locomotor systems because they all use continuous low impact, low stress, and simple movements. This is accompanied by emphasizing rhythmic breathing during full range of movement of the joints. These old traditions, especially the Chinese, advocate daily exercise to avoid stagnation of the chi energy force. In traditional Chinese medicine theories of meridians, acupuncture points, and muscle-tendon continuum, also known as muscle sinews create the concept of a continuum of tissue in the body. Muscle sinews run along the acupuncture meridians, but are wider and more superficial (approx. 1 cm below the skin.) Modern anatomic knowledge suggests that this tissue definition could be a localized area of the deep fascia (Deadman et al., 1998) (Fig. 2.31).

BOX 2.12—**cont'd**

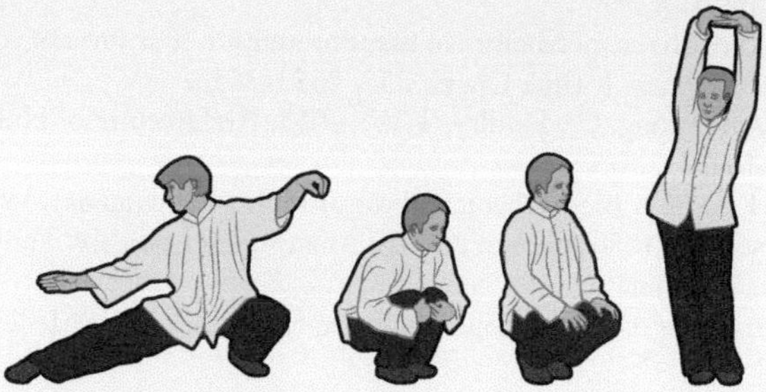

Fig. 2.31 Example of Tai chi exercise.

reinforcements within our fascial system. These phenomena are clearly visible when we study the anatomy of the human body. The way we live our life and the things we have experienced are visible in our body. Our bodies are unique and that's why compensations and dysfunctions can be very variable. For these reasons we need treatment modalities that consider the traumas, operations, and other dysfunctions that occur in our patient's lives. FM converts anatomic knowledge into clinical wisdom.

References

Benetazzo, L., Bizzego, A., De Caro, R., Frigo, G., Guidolin, D., Stecco, C., 2011. 3D reconstruction of the crural and thoracolumbar fasciae. Surg. Radiol. Anat. http://dx.doi.org/10.1007/s00276-010-0757-7.

Benninghoff, A., 1994. Makroskopische Anatomie, Embryologie und Histologie des Menschen. Elsevier. http://dx.doi.org/10.1159/000147570.

Butler, D., 2000. The Sensitive Nervous System. Noigroup Publications, Adelaide, Australia.

Carano, A., Sicialini, G., 1996. Effects of continuous and intermittent forces on human fibroblasts in vitro. Eur. J. Orthod. 18 (1), 19–26.

Chiarugi, G., Bucciante, L., 1975. Istituzioni di Anatomia dell'uomo, 11th ed. Vallardi-Piccin, Padova.

Davies, R.E., 1963. A molecular theory of muscle contraction: calcium-dependent contractions with hydrogen bond formation plus ATP-dependent extensions of part of the myosin-actin cross-bridges. Nature. http://dx.doi.org/10.1038/1991068a.

Deadman, P., Al-Khafaji, M., Baker, K., 1998. A Manual of Acupuncture. Journal of Chinese Medicine Publications. Eastland press. England.

Drake, R., Wayne Vogl, A., Mitchell, A.D.M., 2015. Gray's Anatomy for Students, third ed. Churchill Livingstone.

Federative Committee on Anatomical Terminology, 1998. Terminologia Anatomica.

Findley, T., Chaudry, H., Stecco, A., Roman, M., 2012. Fascia research—A narrative review. J. Bodyw. Mov. Ther. 16 (1), 67–75.

Franklyn-Miller, A., Falvey, E., Clark, R., et al., 2009. The strain patterns of the deep fascia of the lower limb. Fascial Research II: Basic Science and Implications for Conventional and Complementary Health Care. Elsevier.

Gerber, G., 1960. Studies on the metabolism of tissue proteins. 1. Turnover of collagen labeled with prolineTJ-C^{14} in young rats. J. Biol. Chem. 235, 2653–2656.

Guimberteau, J.-C., Armstrong, C., Findley, T.W., 2015. Architecture of Human Living Fascia. Handspring Publishing.

Hamill, J., Knutzen, K., 2009. Biomechanical Basis of Human Movement. Williams & Wilkins.

Jacob, N.H., Bourgery, J.M., 1850. Atlas of Human Anatomy and Surgery. Traité complet de l'anatomie de l'homme. Taschen.

Kannus, P., 2008. Structure of the tendon connective tissue. Scand. J. Med. Sci. Sports 10 (6), 312–320.

Klein, D.M., Katzman, B.M., Mesa, J.A., Lipton, F.L., Caligiuri, D.A., 1999. Histology of the extensor retinaculum of the wrist and the ankle. J. Hand Surg. 24 (4), 799–802.

Knierim, J., 1997. Neuroscience Online an Electronic Textbook for the Neuroscience. University of Texas. http://neuroscience.uth.tmc.edu/s3/index.htm.

Langevin, H., 2006. Connective tissue: a body-wide signaling network? Med. Hypothesis. http://dx.doi.org/10.1016/j.mehy.2005.12.032.

Langevin, H., Fox, J.R., Koptiuch, C., Badger, G.J., Greenan-Naumann, A.C., Bouffard, N.A., et al., 2011. Reduced thoracolumbar fascia shear strain in human chronic low back pain. BMC Musculoskelet. Disord. http://dx.doi.org/10.1186/1471-2474-12-203.

Lieberman, D.E., Raichlen, D.A., Pontzer, H., et al., 2006. The human gluteus maximus and its role in running. J. Exp. Biol. http://dx.doi.org/10.1242/jeb.02255.

Luomala, T., Pihlman, M., Heiskanen, J., Stecco, C., 2014. J. Bodyw. Mov. Ther., 462–468.

Magnusson, S.P., Langberg, H., Kjaer, M., 2010. The pathogenesis of tendinopathy: balancing the response to loading. Nat. Rev. Rheumatol. 6, 262–268.

McCormick, R.J., 1994. The flexibility of the collagen compartment of muscle. Meat Sci. http://dx.doi.org/10.1016/0309-1740(94)90035-3.

Meltzer, K., Cao, T., Schad, J., King, H., Stoll, S., Standley, P., 2010. In vitro modeling of repetitive motion injury and myofascial release. J. Bodyw. Mov. Ther. 14, 162–171.

Müller, W.E.G., 2003. The origin of metazoan complexity: porifera as integrated animals. Integr. Comp. Biol. http://dx.doi.org/10.1093/icb/43.1.3 DOI:10.1093%2Ficb%2F43.1.3.

Powers, C., Chen, Y.-J., Farrokhi, S., Lee, T., 2006. Role of peripatellar retinaculum in transmission of forces within the extensor mechanism. J. Bone Joint Surg. Am. 88 (9), 2042–2048. http://dx.doi.org/10.2106/JBJS.E.00929.

Purslow, P., 2010. Muscle fascia and force transmission. J. Bodyw. Mov. Ther. http://dx.doi.org/10.1016/j.jbmt.2010.01.005.

Reuell, P., 2015. Understanding the IT-Band. http://news.harvard.edu/gazette/story/2015/08/understanding-the-it-band/.

Schilder, A., Hoheisel, U., Magerl, W., Benrath, J., Klein, T., Treede, R.D., 2014. Deep tissue and back pain: stimulation of the thoracolumbar fascia with hypertonic saline. Schmerz. http://dx.doi.org/10.1007/s00482-013-1373-3.

Schleip, R., Müller, D., 2012. Training principals for fascial connective tissue: scientific foundation and suggested practical application. J. Bodyw. Mov. Ther. http://dx.doi.org/10.1016/j.jbmt.2012.06.007.

Schleip, R., Findley, T., Chaitow, L., Huijing, P., 2012. Fascia: The Tensional Network of the Human Body. Churchill Livingstone.

Scott, W., Stevens, J., Binder–Macleod, S.A., 2001. Human skeletal muscle fiber type classification. Phys. Ther. http://ptjournal.apta.org/content/81/11/1810.

Shepherd, J.T., Abboud, F.M., 1977. Handbook of Physiology. Sect 2, Vol. III, Part 2. pp. 623–658.

Siddhartha, S., Shah, J., Gebreab, T., Yen, R.-H., Gilliams, E., Danoff, J., et al., 2009. Novel applications of ultrasound technology to visualize and characterize myofascial trigger points and surrounding soft tissue. Arch. Phys. Med. Rehab. 90, 1829–1838.

Smeulders, M., Kreulen, M., Hage, J., Huijing, P., van der Horst, C., 2005. Spastic muscle properties are affected by length changes of adjacent structures. Muscle Nerve. http://dx.doi.org/10.1002/mus.20360.

Stecco, C., 2015a. Functional Atlas of the Human Fascial System. Churchill Livingstone, Elsevier.

Stecco, C., 2015b. Anatomical Concept of Fascia. Fascial Research IV.

Stecco, C., Schleip, R., 2015. A fascia and the fascial system. J. Bodyw. Mov. Ther. Available from, https://www.researchgate.net/publication/284513539_A_Fascia_and_The_Fascial_System. http://dx.doi.org/10.1016/j.jbmt.2015.11.012.

Stecco, C., Stecco, A., 2012. Deep fascia of the lower limbs. In: Schleip, R., Findley, T., Chaitow, L., Huijing, P. (Eds.), In the book: Fascia – The Tensional Network of the Human Body. Churchill Livingstone Elsevier.

Stecco, L., Stecco, C., 2014. Fascial Manipulation for Internal Dysfunction. Piccin.

Stecco, C., Gagey, O., Belloni, A., et al., 2007. Anatomy of the deep fascia of the upper limb. Second part: study of innervation. Morphologie 91, 38–43.

Stecco, C., Stern, R., Porzionato, A., et al., 2011. Hyaluronan within fascia in the etiology of myofascial pain. Surg. Radiol. Anat. 33, 891–896.

Stecco, A., Wolfgang, G., Robert, H., Fullerton, B., Stecco, C., 2013a. The anatomical and functional relation between gluteus maximus and fascia lata. J. Bodyw. Mov. Ther. 17, 512–517.

Stecco, A., Gesi, M., Stecco, C., Ster, R., 2013b. Fascial components of the myofascial pain syndrome. Curr. Pain Headache Rep. 17, 32.

Stecco, A., Stern, R., Fantoni, I., De Caro, R., Stecco, C., 2015. Fascial disorders: implications for treatment. PM R. http://dx.doi.org/10.1016/j.pmrj.2015.06.006.

Stecco, C., Macchi, V., Porzionato, A., Morra, A., Parenti, A., Stecco, A., et al., 2010. The ankle retinacula: morphological evidence of the proprioceptive role of the fascial system. Cells Tissues Organs. http://dx.doi.org/10.1159/000290225. www.karger.com/cto.

Still, A., 1899. Philosophy of Osteopathy. A.T. Still.

Stilwell, D.L., 1957. Regional variations in the innervation of deep fasciae and aponeuroses. Anat. Rec. 127, 635–653.

Testut, L., 1895. Traité d'Anatomie Humaine—Tome 3. Doin éditeur, Paris.

Tezars, J., Hoheisel, U., Wiedenhöfer, B., Mense, S., 2011. Neuroscience 194, 302–308.

Tortora, G., Derrickson, B., 2011. Principles of anatomy & physiology. Organization, support and movement, and control systems of the human body. 13th edition. John Wiley & Son.

Van der Wal, J., 2009. The architecture of the connective tissue in the musculoskeletal system—an often overlooked functional parameter as to proprioception in the locomotor apparatus. Int. J. Ther. Massage Bodyw. 2 (4), 9–23.

CHAPTER 3

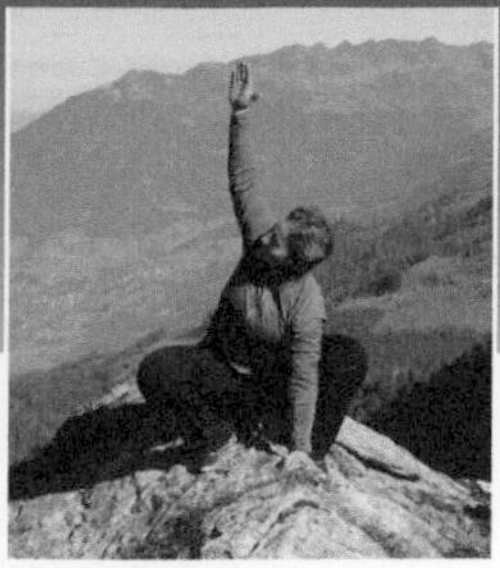

Physiology of the Fascia from the Clinical Point of View

Fascia is associated with many mechanisms in our body and it is easy to visualize it as a form of architecture, like an arch in a cathedral or a bridge that connects an island to a continent (Fig. 3.1). Cars can drive over a bridge from one side to the other; so too fascia can transmit force over short or long distances. These bridges, or fascial layers, are making transportation easier and faster (Fig. 3.2). Deep fascia is responsible for force transmission and proprioception. Loose connective tissue works as a gliding system between the fascial layers and other connective tissue so that proper rigidity and gliding can be achieved. While fascia can function as packing and supporting material for organs and muscles, it is also now considered a sensory organ that communicates with the central nervous system (CNS).

Recent studies have expanded the understanding of the fascial role in vital functions such as the nervous system and the system that controls thermoregulatory and immunologic responses. Subcutaneous tissue, superficial fascia, and the fat tissue above and beneath it form the vital links that are necessary for sensory and immune system functions (Stecco, 2015). Fascial architecture, composition, and form are uniquely adapted to its function within the body and, in the light of this knowledge, fascia is much more than just a piece of architecture.

Fascia and Force Transmission

The many forms of fascia permit its diversity of function. Basically, the constitution, orientation, and consistency of fascia determine its physiologic abilities. The deep fascia consists of aponeurotic and epimysial layers. Aponeurotic fascia slides over epimysial fascia and transmits force over a distance. Epimysial fascia is also capable of force transmission, but over local and shorter distances compared to aponeurotic fascia. Epimysial fascia is thinner than its aponeurotic "big brother" but both are dense connective tissue with a multilayered complex. The biggest difference is that epimysial fascia has tight adherence to the underlying muscles. From the fascial manipulation (FM) point of view aponeurotic fascia is

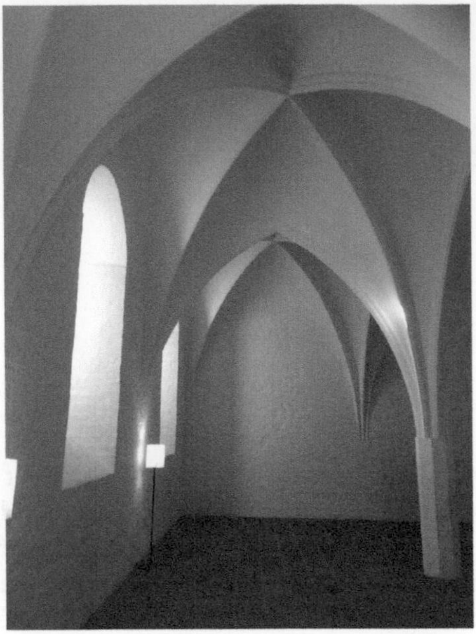

Fig. 3.1 Arch of the Hämeenlinna Castle, Finland.

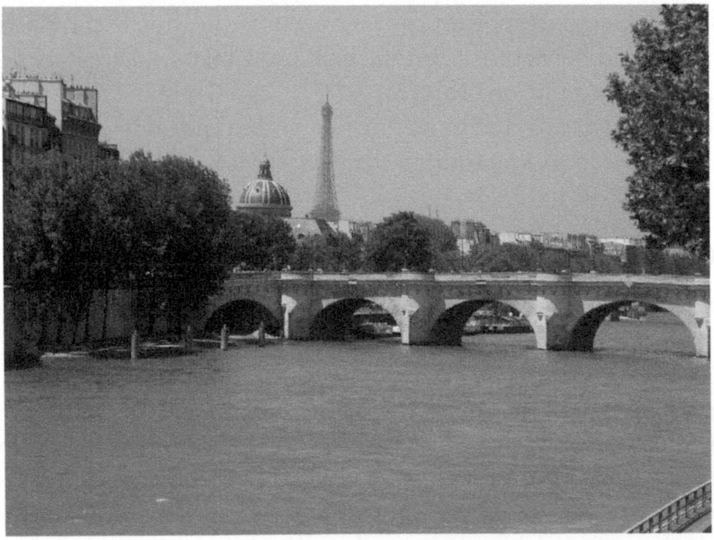

Fig. 3.2 Image of fascial layers as a bridge.

connecting different segments together, and epimysial fascia is transmitting forces related to motor units (muscles). Many researchers have reported similar findings showing that fascia is a force transmitter (Findley et al., 2015; Huijing and Baan, 2008; Patel and Lieber, 1997; Purslow, 2010). The concept of force transmission through synergistic muscle groups and myofascial tissue connectivity is supported also by the study of Cruz-Montecinos et al. (2015).

Aponeurotic fascia is a bridgelike force transmission structure. However, a model with two active muscles and one passive connective tissue link between them is too simplistic to represent the actual function of the fascial system. There is a continuum of elements rather than separate structures. There is no clear point where a muscle ends and a tendon or fascia begins. The muscle is a continuum, a complex in which some parts are red, rich in muscle fibres, and others are more whitish, containing predominantly connective tissue. Luomala et al. (2015) have demonstrated this complex structure in animal studies (Fig. 3.3). Aponeurotic fascia is not a block of connective tissue binding other distinct structures together. There are sublayers in the deep fascia and between them there is loose connective

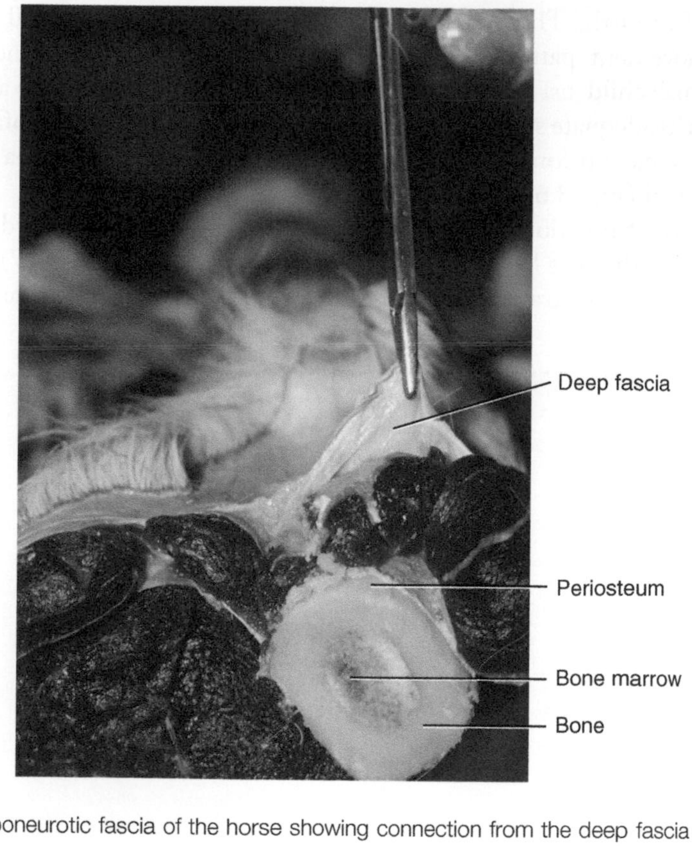

Fig. 3.3 Aponeurotic fascia of the horse showing connection from the deep fascia to the other tissues.

tissue. Thus, when a force is transmitted to an area, aponeurotic fascia adapts to the tension and transmits the force, not only to the nearest contiguous area of the muscle but also to muscles from the opposite side (agonist–antagonist) that are part of its muscular complex. Huijing and Baan (2008) support the hypothesis of the lateral force transmission between the synergists and antagonist muscle via fascial sheaths. This reinforces Luigi Stecco's idea of segments and the meaning of palpation through the whole segment in three dimensions.

This complex system has an important neural component. The deep fascia contains mechanoreceptors sending on-line information about local tension to the CNS. Concurrently with force transmission, the mechanoreceptors in aponeurotic fascia scan for tension variations and with the help of the muscle spindles permit fine, precisely calibrated musculoskeletal movement. Can aponeurotic fascia be likened to a bridge? Yes, but this bridge is very complex and adaptable (Fig. 3.4, Box 3.1).

Collagen reacts to tension. It is designed to bind tissues together and in doing so it will strengthen via tension. A good example is a newborn baby. Connective tissue guides our development in our mother's womb and this development will continue after birth. The evolvement of our myofascial system will continue through movement patterns when we start to move (Marchuk and Stecco, 2015). A small child just learning to stand and bend forward to pick up a toy from the floor lacks adequate stability. At this stage of development the myofascial and nervous systems and force transmission through thoracolumbar fascia have not fully developed (Fig. 3.6).

An important function of the thoracolumbar fascia was emphasized by Serge Gracovetsky at the first Fascia Research Congress (Gracovetsky, 2007). He presented the flexion relaxation phenomenon in healthy backs and discussed the

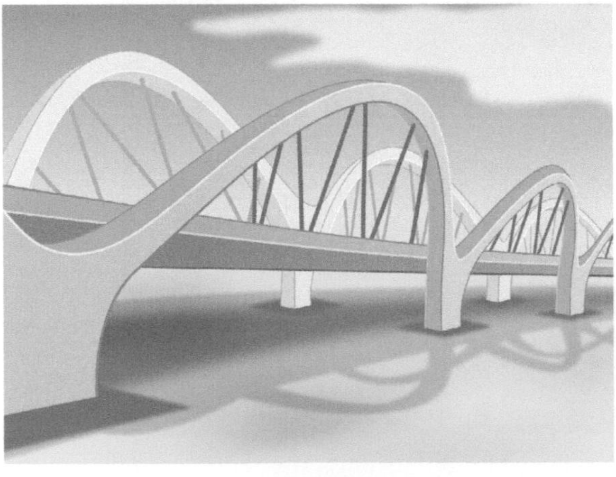

Fig. 3.4 Bridge from the future, complex and adaptable.

BOX 3.1

The thoracolumbar fascia (TLF) represents the deep fascia of the lumbar portion of the back (Fig. 3.5). It has an anterior and a posterior layer, which form a fascial compartment for the erector spinae muscles. Its anterior layer attaches to the tips of the lumbar transverse processes and to the internal oblique and transversus abdominis muscles. The posterior layer attaches to the lumbar supraspinal ligaments and spinous processes to L4, then down to the sacrum, posterior iliac spine, and iliac crest. The posterior fascial layer contains the gluteus maximus and latissimus dorsi muscles, allowing them to function each with different fibre directions along different lines of force. Because of this fascial layer both muscles are allowed to contract simultaneously, allowing connection between the two halves of the body. Vleeming (1995) showed the transfer of forces occurring through this layer from the biceps femoris to the sacrotuberous ligament to the erector spinae to the thoracolumbar fascia to the contralateral latissimus dorsi. The TLF therefore is responsible for the pendulum-like actions of the contralateral arms and legs during walking and running and at the same time acts to stabilize the lower lumbar spine and sacroiliac joints.

Myofascial continuity and expansion are also present in the distal part of the gluteus maximus muscle. Due to its myofascial expansions it can work as a tensioner of the fascia lata together with the tensor fascia latae muscle and other muscles in the thigh area. (Stecco et al., 2013). This ability to transfer force is crucial to human movement. The functions of the fasciae also include tissue proprioception and binding. Because of this, the gluteus maximus muscle is appropriately positioned between the thoracolumbar fascia and the deep fascia of the thigh (fascia lata) to coordinate muscular forces relating to both the lower extremity and torso. Wilke et al. (2015) studied the continuity of the iliotibial tract to the crural fascia and the strong fusion between them was present in every examined subject. This supports the presence of sequences, diagonals, and spirals in our locomotor system.

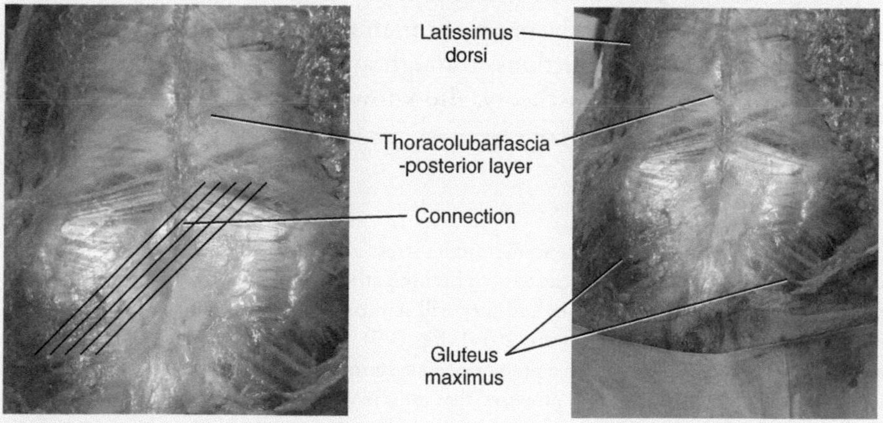

Fig. 3.5 Connection of gluteus maximus and latissimus dorsi through thoracolumbar fascia.

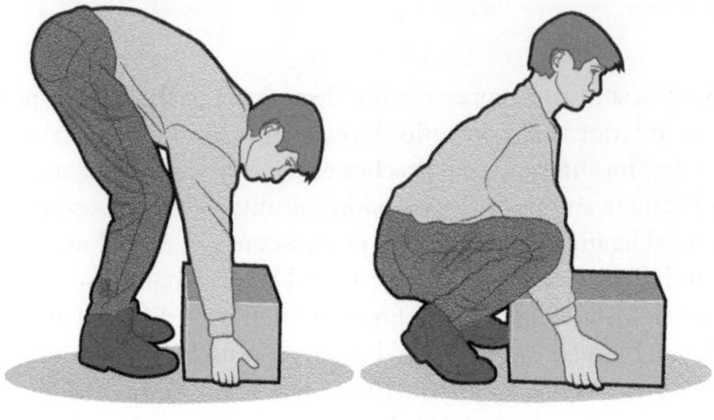

Fig. 3.6 Lifting should be done using multiple methods, sometimes with straight and sometimes bent back to load the fascial system various ways.

erector spinae muscle's potential to extend the back. According to his findings, in flexion of the lumbar spine the erector spinae muscle starts to relax after 20° and the thoracolumbar fascia (TLF) begins to transfer forces from the legs to the torso. At 45° of lumbar flexion the erector spinae is electrically silent (electromyography) and the load is primarily in the fascia. This reaction is reversed if there is back pain due to altered transmission of forces because of possible dysfunction of TLF sublayers sliding past each other. Langevin et al. (2011) studied this hypothesis and found that there are alterations in the connective tissue gliding system in patients with low back pain. We need proper movement between tissues to allow normal force transmission. The restoration of normal gliding between tissues is one of the essential goals of FM (Box 3.2).

The fascial architecture of the muscle from muscle cell to the whole muscle acts to transfer muscular contractions throughout the musculoskeletal system. According to the cross-bridge theory, also known as the sliding filament theory,

BOX 3.2

Most man-made materials become weaker under stress and compression, but under these circumstances, living tissue has the capacity to become stronger. Tissues can resist high strains depending on their size and weight and they will reinforce and become more resistant when stressed gradually (Levin, 2006; Scarr, 2014) (Fig. 3.7). Fascia also acts like a spring, storing and releasing energy. It can act as a pretensioned system allowing the body to function more efficiently. Fukunaga et al. (2002) proposed that muscle work relates more to isometric muscle contraction, while concentric and eccentric action relies more on the elastic component of the myofascial system. The fascial system will get stronger and better orientated under tension. But excessive tension/stress (injury, overuse, surgery) can prevent the fascial system with its sensory elements from functioning normally. For example, mechanoreceptors require a mechanical load of some type to become activated. If they are stuck in nongliding fascia, there will be a failure in mechanoreceptor function. Fascial manipulation helps to solve these problems.

Continued

BOX 3.2—**cont'd**

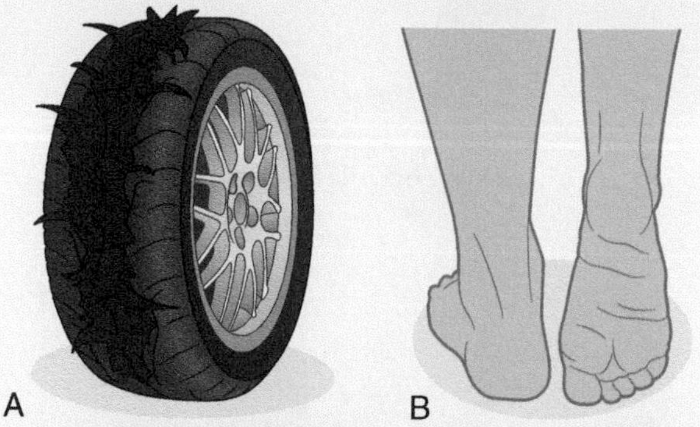

Fig. 3.7 (A) Man-made material such as tyres will become worn when used. (B) Foot sole is getting stronger when loaded progressively. Our tissues need loading to become stronger.

actin and myosin filaments slide past each other creating muscular force, which causes tension in the endomysium (covering of the muscle fibre). When enough fibres are recruited, tension spreads into the perimysium (covering of the muscle bundles), the epimysium (covering of each individual muscle), and finally to the muscle terminations and tendons including myofascial expansions.

Tension is one of the most important features relating to collagen orientation. Tension lines occur in patterns consistent with the orientation of the collagen fibres. Purslow's (2010) study of the endomysium shows the tissue stained, magnified, and clearly visible (Fig. 3.8). There is a contradiction with classic anatomy where force transmission is demonstrated as longitudinal vectors from tendon (origin of the muscle) to tendon (insertion of the muscle). While 70% of the transmission of muscle tension is directed in series through tendons, new information shows that 30% of muscle force is transmitted through the connective structures in parallel, as nonspanning fibres that never reach the tendon (Huijing, 1999; Patel and Lieber, 1997). Some 30% of muscle force is transmitted by the connective tissue (fascia) surrounding the muscle, the deep fascia. The collagen fibres of the endomysium are not longitudinal, but they exist in multidirectional form giving us indications of multidirectional tensions. These findings support Fukunaga's hypothesis (Fukunaga et al., 2002) that human myofibrils contract almost isometrically and concentric "shortening" and eccentric "extending" is more common in connective tissue due to its viscoelastic properties (Fig. 3.9). Whether cells produce longitudinal or multidirectional forces, it is still obvious that muscles are not working as a single unit, but rather as muscle groups working together by way of the fascial system. When we move we use our myofascial system to meet the goals of the movement task.

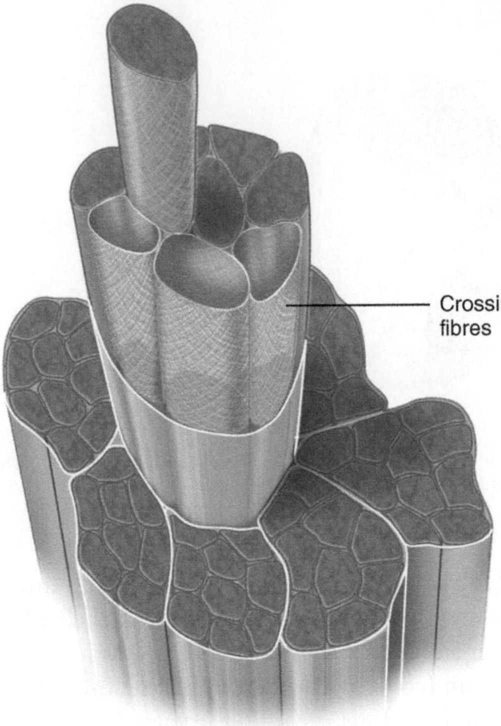

Fig. 3.8 Endomysium is covering the muscle cells. Notice the orientation of the fibres, they are not longitudinal but rather forming a crossing formation to resist the forces and adapt to the activation of the muscle cells.

Fascia participating in mechanotransduction via muscles and the CNS has a crucial role in motor control. The CNS sends electrical impulse signals to the muscle cells, which kick-start the chain reactions in actin and myosin filaments causing a muscle contraction. Those signals start from the motor cortex, travelling via nerve dendrites (motor nerves) to the muscles affecting fascial layers. Nerves perforate finally through the epimysium and continue to the perimysium and terminate at the surface of the muscle cell—the endomysium (Fig. 3.10). Via motor end plates, the signal releases calcium from the sarcoplastic retinaculum causing actin and myosin heads to bind toward each other. The motor unit (alpha motor neuron and muscle cells/fibres it supplies) is the smallest functional unit in the human locomotor system. The amount of motor units varies depending on the amount of fibres it supplies. Each fibre is innervated by a single motor neuron that, according to what is called the innervation number, can activate five fibres for an eye and up to 2000 fibres for a leg. Therefore, fewer units are capable of more precise fine-tuning tasks, such as targeting the eye muscles, while bigger

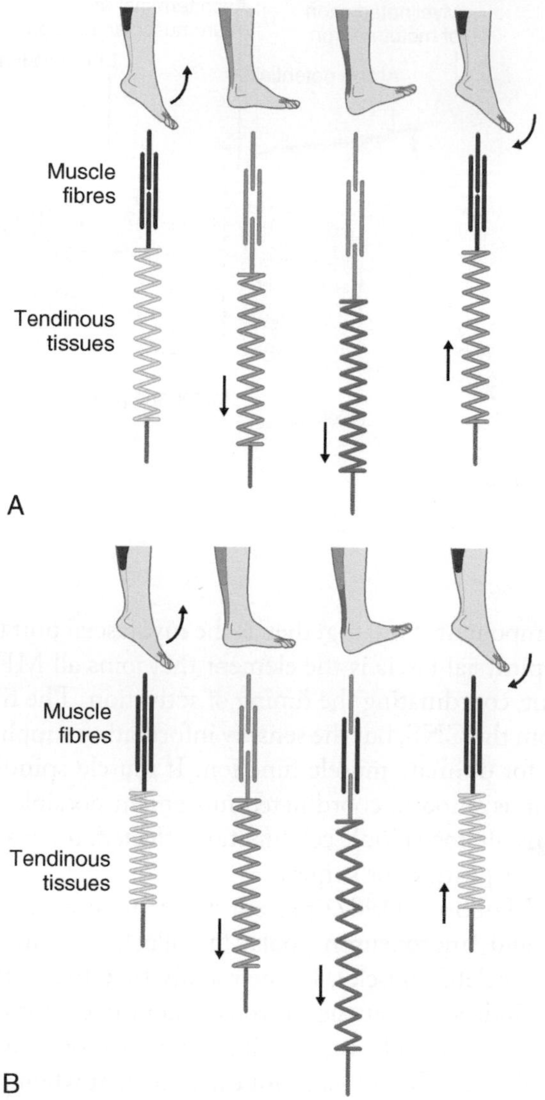

Fig. 3.9 Fukunaga's hypothesis of force transmission assuming that the fascial system would be an important part of the concentric and eccentric loading. (A) Previously thought idea of muscle work. (B) New idea of fascial tissue participation in the movement of the ankle. *(From Schleip and Müller (2013).)*

units (supplying the quadriceps) are for raw and simple tasks like walking. Motor units are an integral part of muscle function. When performing a movement, various motor units of different muscles are usually involved. But to fully understand movement we have to consider more than just muscles. Vascular, neural, bony,

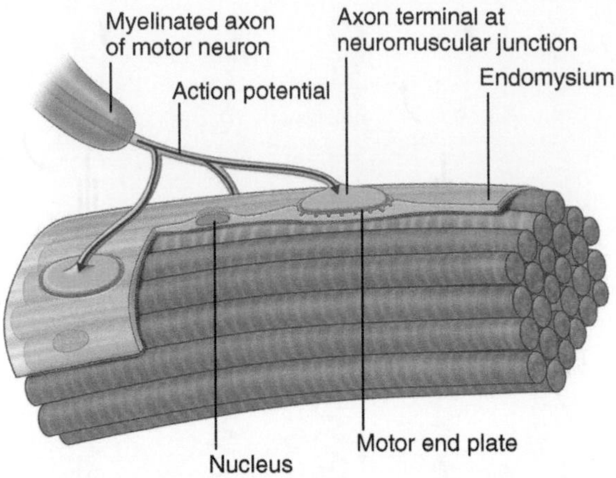

Fig. 3.10 Motor end plate.

and soft tissue components bind together as the myofascial unit (MFU). According to FM, the epimysial fascia is the element that joins all MFUs involved in a specific movement, coordinating the timing of activation. The first input to muscles originates from the CNS, but the sensory information supplied by the spindle cells is necessary for ultimate muscle function. If muscle spindles are tensioned correctly only then is smooth, coordinated movement possible. FM has a direct impact on restoring altered spindle cell function affected, for example, by overuse, injury, trauma, poor posture, or surgery.

De Luca and Mambrito (1987) present an intriguing idea. They discussed "common drive" and "motoneuron pools" (a collection of motor neurons that innervate a single skeletal muscle). In their study they found that the existence of common drive indicates that the nervous system does not control the firing rates of motor units individually. Instead, it acts on the motoneuron pool in a uniform fashion. Applied to FM it means, for example, that when part of the deltoid muscle contracts, it will stretch the perimysium of the brachial muscle where the muscle spindles are present. Consequently, this stretching activates the muscle spindle and the myotatic reflex, causing the contraction of the extrafusal muscular fibres of the brachialis muscle (in this case, only those fibres connected with the deltoid muscle and related fascia). This is an example of peripheral motor coordination that permits the coactivation of deltoid and brachialis and their fascia. This kind of complex regulation fits perfectly with the fascia's ability to bind and its rich and dense innervation. It seems that human anatomic function is much more complex than just muscle pairs forming force partners that work via an on–off system (Box 3.3).

BOX 3.3 Fascial Continuum and Muscle Function

Myofascial continuums are present throughout our body. The deltoid and brachialis muscles are good examples of the fascial continuum system. With this example we can contemplate how muscles are working and how they are organized. The deltoid is an interesting muscle as it is attached proximally to the clavicle, acromion, and spine of scapula. Distally it is inserted to the deltoid tuberosity. Pihlman et al. (2015) demonstrated that the insertion of the deltoid is not as clear as it seems. There is a tendon travelling to the deltoid tuberosity, but mostly from the anterior portion of the deltoid. The lateral and posterior parts of the deltoid have strong horizontal muscle fibre alignment suggesting rotational force generation. These parts travel over the deltoid tuberosity and insert directly into the brachialis muscle. With ultrasonography imaging we can distinguish a very clear continuum between muscle fibres and the fascial continuum that creates a bridgelike connection between muscles (Fig. 3.11).

The function of this coupled system is interesting. The deltoid muscle lies over the shoulder joint (glenohumeral) which is a ball-and-socket joint. This joint moves in all anatomic planes and combinations of planes. The muscle bulk is located in front of the shoulder, on the lateral side of the shoulder, and behind it. For that reason it acts as the shoulder joint's flexor, extensor, abductor, internal, and external rotator. Actually the deltoid creates its own agonist–antagonist force couple. In this way the deltoid creates its own counterforce. This is contradictory to the general biomechanical principle that posits that two or more muscles are needed to create an antagonistic force. One muscle extends and another flexes. From the fascial point of view this unity follows the idea of lateral force transmission and balancing of the sequences in fascial manipulation treatment.

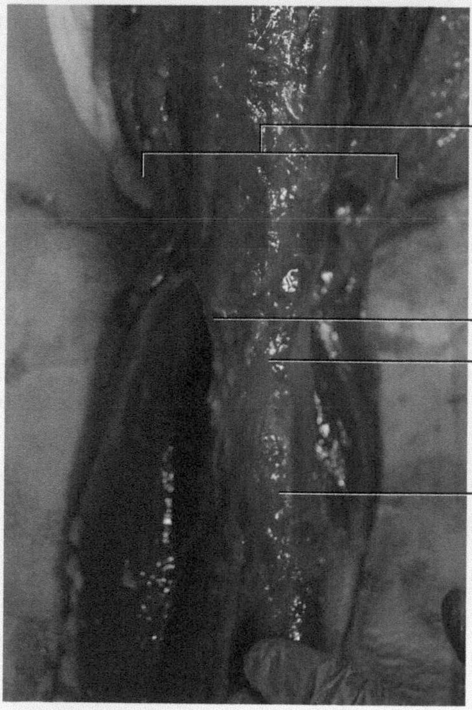

Fig. 3.11 Continuum of deltoid and brachialis muscles with fascial and muscular attachments.

Myofascial Expansions

"The term myofascial expansion indicates each connection that originates from a skeletal muscle, or from its tendon, inserting into the aponeurotic fascia." (Stecco C., 2015; Box 3.4).

Definitions of myofascial expansion (MFE) have also been described or proposed by others from Chiarugi and Bucciante (1975) to Standring (2008). Similar descriptions are found in Da Vinci's famous writings over 500 years ago where he described deltoid muscle anatomy as "which part insert to bone and which are inserted to other muscles." MFE refers to all anatomic connections from muscle tissue (myo) to deep fascia (fascial) and not just to muscle–fascia links, but to all links between muscles. Those links are often present in tendon areas, where the tendon inserts into bone. Tendons are covered with fascial sheets, which are expanding the insertional area to a wider area, not only to one spot. No longer is it correct to define muscle attachments by way of singular origins and insertions. Perhaps the most famous expansion is the lacertus fibrosus, which arise from biceps brachii muscles' insertional tendon to cover flexor muscles of the wrist. (antebrachial fascia–deep fascia of the forearm). In Fig. 3.12, myofascial expansion, lacertus fibrosus, and antebrachial fascia are illustrated. When looking carefully, similar expansions can be found hidden behind the lacertus fibrosus. The brachialis and biceps are not exceptions since almost all muscles have similar expansions. For example, the quadriceps not only inserts into the tibial tuberosity but also expands to the anterior retinaculum of the knee. It expands to the lateral side of knee, tractus iliotibialis, and medially to the pes anserinus. The gluteus maximus has numerous expansions, some proximal, attaching to the crista iliaca and sacrum and then on to the trunk via the thoracolumbar fascia. Distally the gluteus maximus inserts into the femur (tuberosity of glutei), with most of its

BOX 3.4

Almost all muscles and tendons connect to what are called myofascial expansions. An obvious expansion is the thickened lacertus fibrosis that originates from the biceps brachii tendon and merges with the antebrachial fascia. Carla Stecco (2015) gives four examples of myofascial expansions:

1. muscle fibres that originate directly from fascia,
2. muscle fibres that insert into fascia,
3. tendinous expansions that originate from facia, and
4. tendinous expansions that insert into fascia.

When muscles contract they stretch the surrounding fascia and the myofascial expansions, both of which contain the sensory receptors necessary for proper muscle function and coordination.

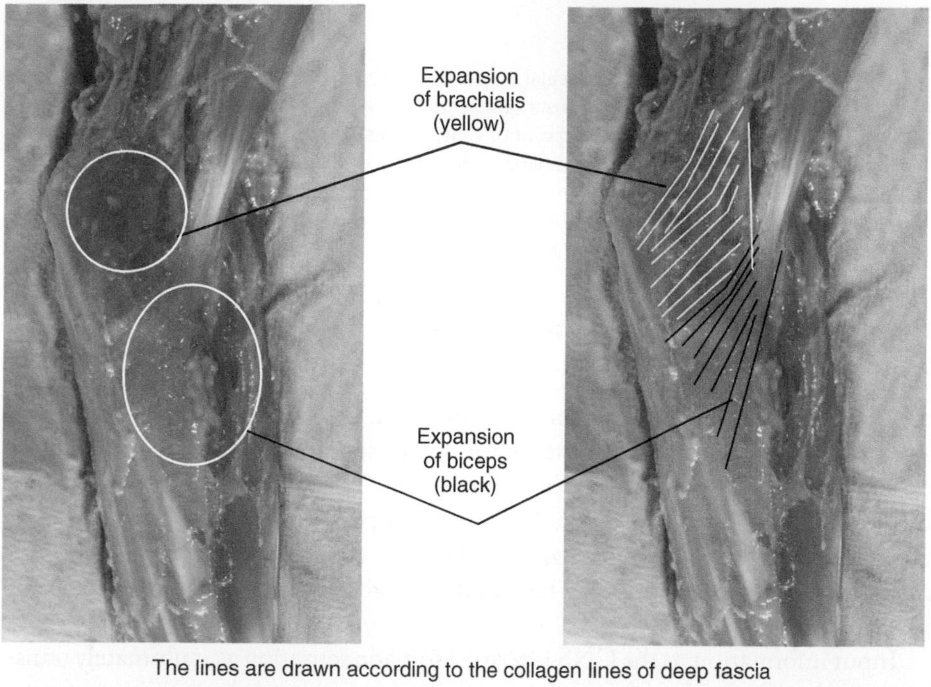

Fig. 3.12 Myofascial expansion of lacertus fibrosus originating from biceps brachii and expansion of brachialis under the lacertus fibrosus.

fibres traveling to the deep fascia of the thigh (fascia lata), and into the tractus iliotibialis that inserts laterally below the knee.

Muscles have been defined by ancient cultural and historical traditions. Our way of understanding anatomy originates from ancient Egypt, Greek, and Roman eras. The University of Padua has had a great influence since the Middle Ages, and now Carla Stecco (Stecco, 2015) writes and expands on the function and anatomy of fascia. Every muscle contraction automatically stretches its fascial expansions. Imagine a tent and its canvas tensioned by ropes, poles, or sticks as an example of the MFE. Deep fascia is the canvas covering the limbs, trunk, and bones. Muscles can be seen as the sticks and ropes that create tension in the tent. Expansions create stretch into deep fascia and they transfer strength and tension over a distance during muscle contraction. Muscle contraction selectively stretches the portions of the deep fascia via the MFE. Mechanoreceptors located in the deep fascia are stimulated when stretched sending proprioceptive feedback to the CNS. This reciprocal information between the myofascial system and the CNS is essential for normal feedback regarding all movements (Box 3.5).

BOX 3.5

Myofascial expansions transfer muscular forces over a distance and at the same time create stretch to the deep fascia. This allows our central nervous system to detect proprioceptive feedback. From the fascial manipulation point of view, expansions are crucial for the formation of the tensional points (centres of coordination and centres of fusion) into line-based networks. The myofascial relation between muscles and the proprioceptive system "underlines the peripheral coordination among the various muscles involved in the movement and perception of correct motor direction" (Stecco, 2015).

Proprioceptive Role of the Fascia

In the nervous system, all impulses of the "input system" flow toward the spinal cord and finally to the sensory cortex of the brain. Information is processed in the sensory cortex and from there the motor nerves send orders to the target tissues. Sensory information is gathered by the receptors. There are different receptors for different tasks. Thermoreceptors fire when temperature changes and mechanoreceptors fire when some mechanical alteration occurs, pressure or tension, for instance. Mechanoreceptors can be found throughout the human body, especially in the deep fascia.

Input information to the CNS is termed somatic sensation as it ultimately transmits touch, pressure, length and degree of stretch, tension, and contraction of muscles to the brain. This information system also interprets sensory information from temperature and joint position as well as nociception from free nerve endings. The central and peripheral nervous systems are coordinated to receive and interpret sensory information from organs, joints, ligaments, muscles, fascia, and skin (Box 3.6). Mechanical changes are part of a somatic sensation that stimulates mechanoreceptors (Tortora and Derrickson, 2011). Because of the density of nerves and its broad innervation, fascia has a marked ability to sense changes in the tissues including the joints. Small movements of the joints will not stretch a capsule, but will cause a change in tension at the deep fascial level. This will launch mechanoreceptors, which send impulses to the CNS. Keeping this in mind, we can imagine a cobweb and a spider in it. The web is the fascia covering the tissues. The spider is the CNS that uses the web to feel even the smallest vibrations, which are signs that something has been caught to be eaten at dinner time. (Fig. 3.13).

BOX 3.6

Skin is usually thought to be our most sensitive organ, but many researchers have found similar receptors in deep fascia. These findings indicate that the deep fascia is highly innervated like retinacula and skin. Thus, fascia serves as a bodywide mechanosensitive signalling system and there is no doubt that fascial structures play an important role in proprioception (Benjamin, 2009; Langevin, 2006; Stecco et al., 2007, Tezars et al., 2011).

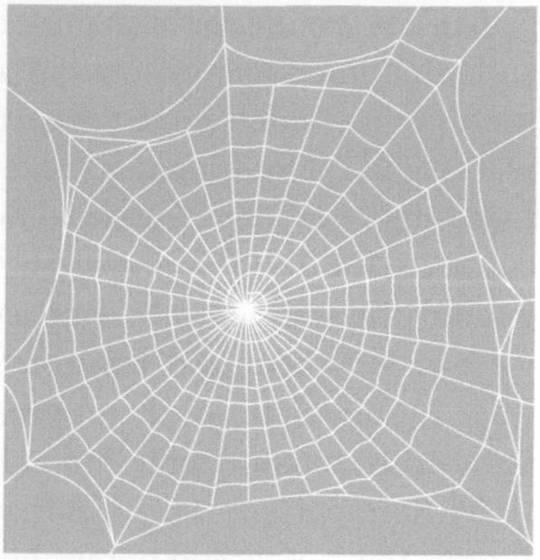

Fig. 3.13 Image of a spider web. Fascia can be thought of as a spider web where vibrations are travelling through the whole web.

In FM, Golgi tendon organs (GTOs) are fundamental in regulating the equilibrium between the agonist and antagonist muscles. GTOs are located in the junction between skeletal muscle fibres and tendon where they are surrounded by collagen fibre bundles. When the collagen fibres are stretched, the GTO reacts and fires an impulse along the input sensory system. The GTO continuously measures the force in a contracting muscle. The job of the GTO is to determine how tense or relaxed a muscle is by sending information to the spinal cord. The CNS will either let the muscle continue to work or send an order to the muscle to relax. When a leg "gives way" suddenly during walking, the cause could be a misfiring of the GTO. Most misfired GTOs result from myofascial dysfunction that has caused an oversensitivity to its receptors. In rehabilitation, GTOs have also been used by PNF stretching (Adler et al., 2008) contract–relax application (Fig. 3.14).

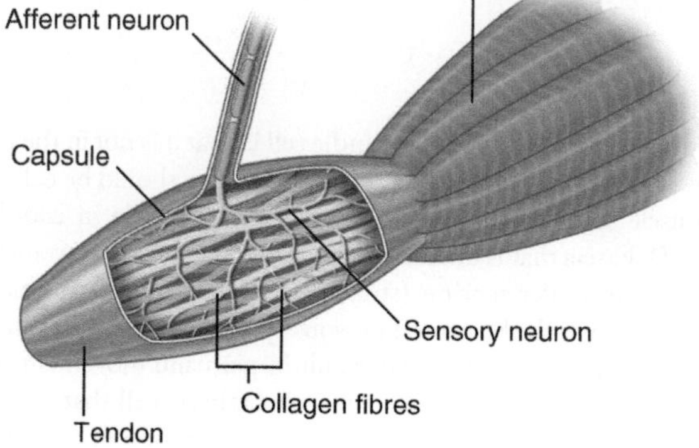

Fig. 3.14 Golgi tendon organs(GTO) are surrounded by collagen fibre bundles located in the junction between muscle fibres and tendons.

Muscle spindles have an important role in FM treatment. They have excitation and inhibition force-generating properties. This system can activate or shut down motor units, which are either necessary or useless. In this way, muscle spindles are working like light dimmers. They can control how much light you will have in the room, more or less. Muscle spindles are inside the muscle and they are strongly connected to the fascial system like electrical wires in our houses are travelling behind the walls closely connected to the wall. Switches are the places where we can see them and control the system by using the dimmers in a proper way. Intrafusal fibres themselves are part of the continuum and they are constructed from contractile muscular fibres within a fascial component.

Most important is the fact that the muscle spindle is within the fascia that surrounds the muscle and not in the muscle itself. As Carla Stecco states in her book (2015) muscle spindle cells should be more appropriately called "fascial spindle cells." Tension of the epimysium, perimysium, and endomysium can affect the function of the muscle spindle. Abnormal tension can create dysfunction in the force generation system via fascial layers. Because spindles adhere to intramuscular fascia, fascial dysfunctions can alter the normal function of the spindles (Box 3.7). Tensional changes in the fascial system can alter the spindle cell ability to react and therefore may lead to motor control dysfunction, for example, changes in the input system leading to changes in strength output. Because many of these receptors lie mostly in fascia, fascial dysfunction can alter information or at least corrupt it.

Role of the Fascia in Pain Perception

A series of recent reports address the possible involvement of the deep fascia in myofascial pain (Stecco et al., 2013). Variations in deep fascia thickness occur in subjects with chronic low back pain (Langevin et al., 2011) or chronic neck pain (Stecco et al., 2014). The ingrowth of nociceptive fibres and immunoreactions to

BOX 3.7

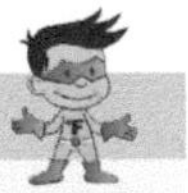

The most important point about this muscle spindle cell is that it is not in the muscle but in the fascia as stated above. As Stecco (2015) states in her text, they should be called fascial spindle cells rather than muscle spindle cells. Muscle spindles have a role in coordinating specific motor units (Fig. 3.15). Fascia that is unable to glide prevents normal movement of the spindle cells, which have to be to under tension (stretch) during a muscle contraction. Failure of spindle cell communication with the central nervous system results in dysfunction and compensations in the myofascial system. This will result in pain and movement disorder. One of the main effects of fascial manipulation is to allow the spindle cell that is stuck in densified fascia to be allowed to glide. Restoration of normal proprioception in the human and animal body allows normal muscle coordination to occur. With uncoordinated fascia, there will be pain, stiffness, and an increase in recidivism of past injuries.

Continued

BOX 3.7—cont'd

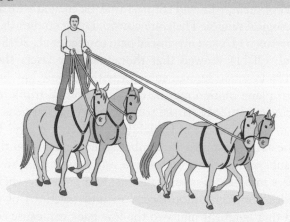

Fig. 3.15 Muscle spindle imaged as a rider handling many horses at the same time. The rider is a muscle spindle that is controlling the activated muscle cells (horses).

substance P have been found in the loose connective tissue of the deep fascia (retinaculum) of patients with patella–femoral alignment problems (Sanchis-Alfonso and Rosello-Sastre, 2000), while a loss of nerve fibres in the thoracolumbar fascia has been reported in patients with chronic lumbago (Bednar et al., 1995). Innervation of the thoracolumbar fascia by both A-fibre and C-fibre nociceptors has been suggested by long-lasting sensitization of the deep fascia in response to mechanical pressure and chemical stimulation (Deising et al., 2012; Schilder et al., 2014). Interestingly, the same authors demonstrate that the sensitized free nerve fibre endings within muscle fascia are stimulated more effectively when the fascia is "prestretched" by muscle contraction.

It is possible that the viscoelasticity of fascia can modify activation of the proprioceptors within fascia. Indeed, the free nerve endings and the proprioceptive corpuscles are completely embedded inside the fascia. If the deep fascia is overstretched, or if it becomes too viscous, it is probable that the nerves inside the fascia will be activated incorrectly. The concept of gliding within the fascial system is crucial for normal fascial function. Normal gliding between the layers of fascia surrounding the muscle and within the muscle depends on the normal hydration provided principally by hyaluronan (HA). HA is already proving successful when it is injected into osteoarthritic knees or frozen shoulders. If the HA assumes a more packed conformation, or more generally, if the loose connective tissue inside the fascia alters its density, the behaviour of the entire deep fascia and the underlying muscle would be compromised. This, we predict, may be the basis of the common phenomenon known as myofascial pain. There is evidence that if the loose connective tissue within the fascia has increased viscosity, the receptors will not be activated properly. Densified HA also alters the distribution of the lines of force within the fascia. In this environment, pain and stiffness may be created with stretching even within the physiological ranges. There are corroborating studies that demonstrate the relationship between HA and myofascial pain (Stecco et al., 2013) (see Video 7).

Langevin et al. (2011) showed that thoracolumbar fascia shear strain was approximately 20% lower in human subjects with chronic low back pain. This reduction of shear plane motion may be due to abnormal trunk movement patterns and/or intrinsic connective tissue pathology. What happens if information to the CNS is corrupted because of fascial dysfunction or injury? Panjabi (1992) explained that the ability to move the lumbar spine depends on three individual but cooperating subsystems: the neural, active, and passive subsystems. The active subsystem includes muscles, passive ligaments, and tendons, whereas the neural subsystem includes peripheral proprioception and reactions of CNS. Panjabi (2006) theorized that ligament injury to the low back can cause corrupted feedback to the CNS, which distorts the input–output system. He posited that corrupted feedback changes the motor cortex's ability to produce movement or to hold posture. At the very least, corrupted information affects the quality of those tasks. Since fascial layers are more richly innervated than ligaments, feedback from the fascial layers can also be altered. Fascial tissue is the most richly innervated in the musculoskeletal system so it follows that fascial dysfunction might be crucial to the motor control system. Peripheral alteration can cause changes in the CNS (spinal reflex and cortex of the brain) (Fig. 3.16).

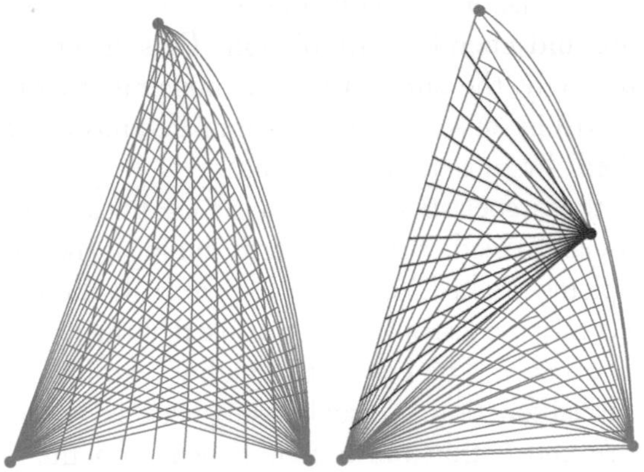

- Standard point of adhesion
- Standard lines of forces inside the deep fascia
- New point of adhesion
- New lines of force

Fig. 3.16 Alteration of the lines of force can change feedback between the tissues and central nervous system. *(From Stecco, 2013.)*

If the tensional system is impaired, fascial dysfunction might create excessive local compression and under prolonged stress it might tear collagen fibres. Schilder et al. (2014) demonstrated that fascia is the most pain-sensitive deep tissue in the low back and can cause widespread referred pain. Besides, fascia as a complex network can also interfere with the mechanics of the nerve by altering the gliding movement of its surrounding fascial layers. For all these reasons, many cases of referred pain like sciatica can be solved by using FM (Box 3.8).

FM always focuses on the history, including injuries and other events. Often "silent" points, that is, not currently exhibiting pain, can be the source of the

BOX 3.8

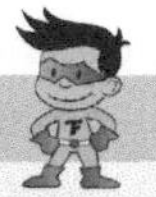

Disc problems have also been under magnification. Jensen et al. (1994) stated that there is a poor correlation between symptoms and magnetic resonance imaging (MRI). He found a lot of disc problems in subjects without low back pain: 64% of nonsymptomatic subjects had intervertebral disc abnormalities and 38% had abnormalities in more than one level. Patients suffering with low back pain often are alarmed at X-ray findings that are totally unrelated to their pain. Disc prolapse or bulge sounds terrifying. Often these patients are complaining of sciatic problems unilaterally. Sciatica is a typical example of referred pain that is thought to be arising from the disc or nerve root. Clinically with fascial manipulation, many cases of sciatic pain can be alleviated by treating the deep fascia of the inferior limbs. Indeed the pain could be due to an overstretching of these fasciae, which chronically stimulate the local nerve receptors (Fig. 3.17).

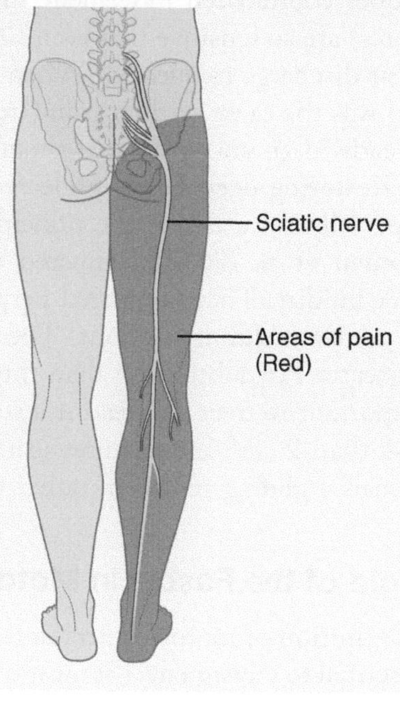

Fig. 3.17 Typical area of sciatic referral. *(From the fascial point of view alteration of the gliding between the fascial layers can cause impairment also to the neural component.)*

problem causing pain along a particular fascial sequence. Compensations are always present in our body and can protect us from experiencing pain. But when compensations are under excess stress we begin to feel discomfort and pain on movement. History of past trauma, posture, and individual movement patterns create unique compensations for every individual. Palpation skills of the therapist are crucial when seeking the origin of the problem. Also precise history-taking will help the decision-making when solving the puzzle of dysfunction.

A second element that can cause pain is due to the strong relationship between muscle spindles and fascia. Indeed if the fascia is altered, the spindle cells may not function normally, depriving the CNS of necessary information about joint movement, muscle coordination, and position. Spindle cells represent a common final pathway since all proprioceptive input from fascia, ligaments, skin, etc., goes to the dorsal horn. The dorsal horn has collaterals that synapse on the gamma motor neurons causing reflex activation of spindle cells. Spindle cells are active even during sleep and they must be stretched during muscle contraction or passively stretched to become activated. It is therefore probable that if the spindle cells are embedded in thickened, densified fascia, their ability to be stretched would be affected and normal spindle cell feedback to the CNS would be altered.

Siegfried Mense, MD, one of the world's leading experts on muscle pain and neurophysiology, when questioned about fascial adhesions having an adverse effect on spindle cells, answered "Structural disorders of the fascia can surely distort the information sent by the spindles to the CNS and thus can interfere with a proper coordinated movement." He added "The primary spindle afferents (Ia fibres) are so sensitive that even slight distortions of the perimysium will change their discharge frequency." When our patients complain that the last thing they did was the cause of their pain ("must have gotten out of bed wrong") they were already in an uncoordinated situation.

Restoring deep fascial glide requires a method of reaching the deep fascia, especially since this is the principal location of the spindle cells and the HA. Roman et al. (2013) compared the methods of manual effects on restoring HA fluidity. They compared perpendicular vibration and tangential oscillation to constant sliding motions. The perpendicular and tangential motions caused a greater HA lubrication than the sliding method. This demonstrates why it is important to treat an area for a sufficient length of time. The treatment area is less than 2 cm^2 and requires usually between 2 and 4 minutes until palpation reveals a gliding sensation rather than a densification (Box 3.9).

Role of the Fascia in Motor Coordination

"Definition of motor control is the ability to regulate or direct the mechanisms essential to movement" (Shumway-Cook and Woollacott, 2007). In other words, motor control refers to the ability to produce and orchestrate bodily movement

BOX 3.9 (see Video 8)

One incidence of dysfunction of motor control can be detected in the areolar tissue, which is the loose connective tissue between the deep fascial layers. Abnormal tension caused by altered fascial gliding will affect the mechanoreceptors, which send false signals to the central nervous system or, in other words, corrupted feedback to the brain. Mechanoreceptors can be sensitized or lose their ability to react depending on the dysfunction in question. Increase in the viscoelastic properties of loose connective tissue could be the result of misuse, disuse, overuse, or trauma (Fig. 3.18). Emotional stress can also create elevated levels of tension in the myofascial system and lead indirectly toward overuse or misuse. For example, the TMJ area (the joint between the temporalis and mandibular bones and the fascia and muscles covering it) seems to be very vulnerable to stress-related dysfunction.

Fascial manipulation rationalizes that stiffness and dysfunction between fascial layers are caused by molecular changes in hyaluronic acid. Hyaluronic acid (HA) allows the fascial layers to slide. Trauma, overuse, and surgery can increase the viscosity of loose connective tissue resulting in tissue changes causing pain or movement dysfunction. A principal reason for fascial dysfunction relates to modification in the properties of HA causing it to change from a sol to gel. HA forms chain links, which cause the extracellular matrix to stiffen. With fascial manipulation we break the cross bridges of HA molecules that change the properties of HA back to the fluid state. In this way abnormal tension in the myofascial web can be released allowing the restricted mechanoreceptors and proprioceptors to function normally.

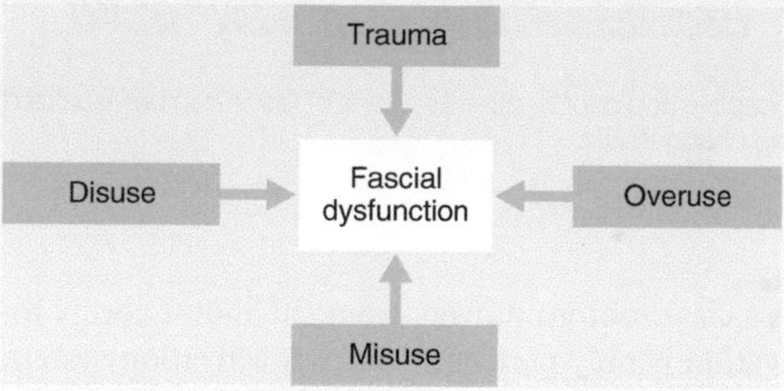

Fig. 3.18 Source of fascial dysfunctions.

over the full range of joint motion in all conditions of intensity and velocity. There is also the consideration of adapting and compensating to physical tasks and the environment at any given moment. Gait is a good example. It is a basic human movement that is performed at a range of velocities from slow (walking) to high (running). In addition, environmental factors like load bearing or the slope of the movement plain will change how the movement is coordinated. The quality of the movement plain, such as uneven ground or rocks, holes, or stairs, will also alter coordination. In addition, the gait task will change if changes occur, like slipping, that require reaction and readjustment. The whole myofascial system is sending and receiving signals when we are moving (Box 3.10).

BOX 3.10

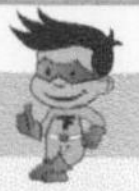

Functions of the motor unit cannot be understood without comprehending fascia and muscle spindles. Muscle spindles are embedded in the epimysium/perimysium along with other mechanoreceptors in the deep fascia. Functionally deep fascia is an important contributor to coordination and proprioception similar to radar (Fig. 3.19). Muscle activation will stretch the perimysium and this will affect muscle spindles. Golgi tendon organs located in the tendon areas will react to the changes in the myofascial tissues. These roles determine fascia's importance in motor control and highlight the importance of proper gliding mechanisms.

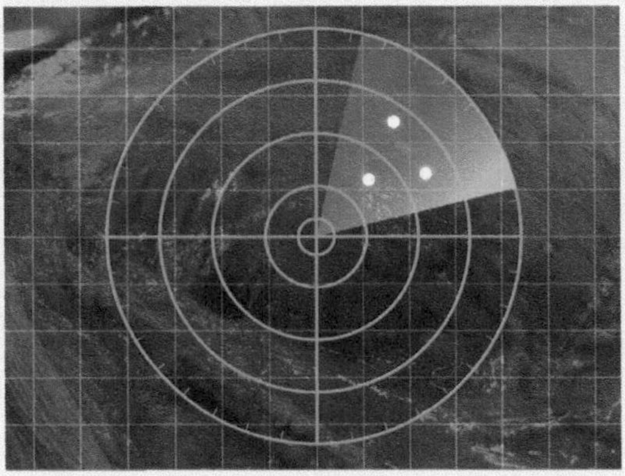

Fig. 3.19 Proprioceptive and coordinative functions of fascia can be visualized as radar scanning the tissue and changes in it.

Thus, there is a clear motor pathway from the motor cortex to the motor end plates. This activation is only part of a complex activation system of the human musculoskeletal system. Conscious actions of the brain are too slow for rapid movements, which are needed in our daily tasks; therefore reflexes play an important role in motor activation. According to Luigi Stecco (Stecco and Stecco, 2009), the fascia is stressed very specifically when motor units are involved in a particular movement. The training reinforces these connections, facilitating the coactivation of a defined movement pattern. So the organization of the deep fascia becomes a key element in peripheral motor control.

Fascia as an Energy Storage

Most of the studies about the elasticity of deep fascia consider the aponeurotic fascial layer. Collagen fibrils cannot be taut. At least some elasticity must be present to permit movement. Tendons, for instance, have the potential to be stretched approximately 3% to 4% (Ker, 1999). In animal tests, the Achilles tendon has the capacity for a 7-mm elongation of its mean length of 180 mm

(Fukunaga et al., 2002; Rosso et al., 2012). Applying this to the human anatomy, the Achilles tendon would have an estimated 4% elasticity. According to Maganaris and Paul (1999) the tibialis anterior (TA) tendon seems to have approximately 2.5% elasticity with electrical stimulus of the TA muscle. Elastic properties are exhibited in two ways: during active contraction of the muscle and passively when mechanical loading is applied. Tendons, ligaments, and deep fascia contain elastin and other elements, which determine the tissue's overall elasticity. Elastin is responsible for most of the elastic capacity together with local fluid changes.

According to Schleip (2003) the interstitial receptors (free nerve endings) make up the majority of sensory input from myofascial tissue and from the autonomic nervous system. The activation of these receptors triggers the autonomic nervous system to change the local pressure in fascial arterioles and capillaries, which in turn causes changes in local fluid dynamics. This changes the tissue's elastic capacity. Studies are needed to yield precise knowledge about the elastic properties of the deep fascia. Studying fresh horse cadavers, Luomala et al. (2015) found that deep fascia elasticity varies from individual to individual in animal studies. Elastic properties of deep fascia from the resting position to the most elongated position caused an elongation of between 10% and 20%. Thirty minutes of continued stretching produced no additional elongation. This suggests that, like tendons and ligaments, deep fascia is elastic but not stretchable after it reaches its limit (Stecco C., 2015) (Fig. 3.20).

In addition to elasticity, many factors contribute to the capacity for movement. Tissues are moving in relationship with each other and different levels of elasticity are present in fascia. The loose connective tissue provides a flexible layer between

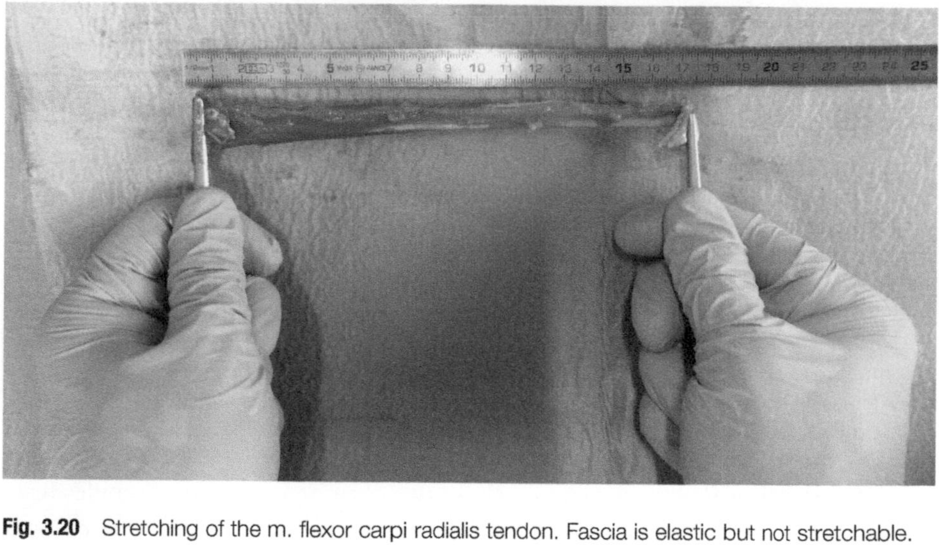

Fig. 3.20 Stretching of the m. flexor carpi radialis tendon. Fascia is elastic but not stretchable.

layers of dense connective tissue that allows structures to move relative to one another. It both promotes movement and contains or limits movement (Benjamin, 2009). This elasticity is important because of elastic energy storage and fascial recoil. We can create similar effects by using FM. Enhancement of the sliding potential will increase the body's capacity to load and reload.

All soft tissue is elastic to some degree. This elasticity allows movement and affects how efficiently tissues produce movement, absorb stress, and tolerate strain. All soft tissue, including collagen, has at least some ability to store mechanical energy. The most simplified assumptions posit that the more the collagen, the stiffer the tissues. Stiffer tissues tolerate stress and store energy better. On the other hand, less collagen yields looser tissue, more lost energy, and less stress and strain absorption. This is the case in hypermobility syndrome (HMS; Box 3.11).

Elastic tissue elongates under load. This elongation stretches the collagen and other elastic elements of the tissue. Storage of elastic energy increases as tissue lengthens. If the stress load is greater than tissue can tolerate, it will tear or rupture. Under normal conditions, the human input–output system will regulate a tissue's stress and force generation. This system will provide feedback (pain) when there is too much load on the musculoskeletal system and often reflex action will stop the movement before tissue damage can occur. Stored energy will be used to produce the next movement. This system permits energy saving and movement

BOX 3.11

Hypermobility syndrome (HMS) is often thought to be a problem in young girls with hyperextended joints. HMS however has been observed in both sexes at every stage of life and in all races. Importantly, HMS is not only a problem of hypermobile joints, it is a systemic disorder related to the connective tissue. Moreover it is connected to the proprioceptive and force transmission properties of the myofascial system. HMS patients present with loose or hyperelastic connective tissue throughout the body: joints, fascia, the entire neurovascular system, and the tissue surrounding the internal organs. Because of the looser tissue, energy storage and reuse is a problem. Therefore HMS patients tend to become overfatigued more often. They may suffer from more overuse-related syndromes and even from difficulty in lifting loads that others feel are lightweight. Higher than expected subluxations, hernias, ruptures, and slow injury recovery may also characterize the HMS patient. Also many HMS patients complain of problems in motor coordination and proprioception. They are twisting joints into awkward positions to have some kind of feeling of normal posture. A sense of the sitting or standing postures is altered. These problems can interfere with daily activities of living, school, or work. The pain associated with HMS can become widespread and persistent and might initially be confused with fibromyalgia. HMS can be diagnosed using Beighton's criteria where Beighton's scoring system is added to other major and minor criteria. Beighton's scoring is not reliable by itself or in children under 13 years (Grahame, 2000). From the FM point of view the therapist has multiple ways to help these patients who are often overlooked and misunderstood (Figs. 3.21 and 3.22).

Continued

BOX 3.11—cont'd

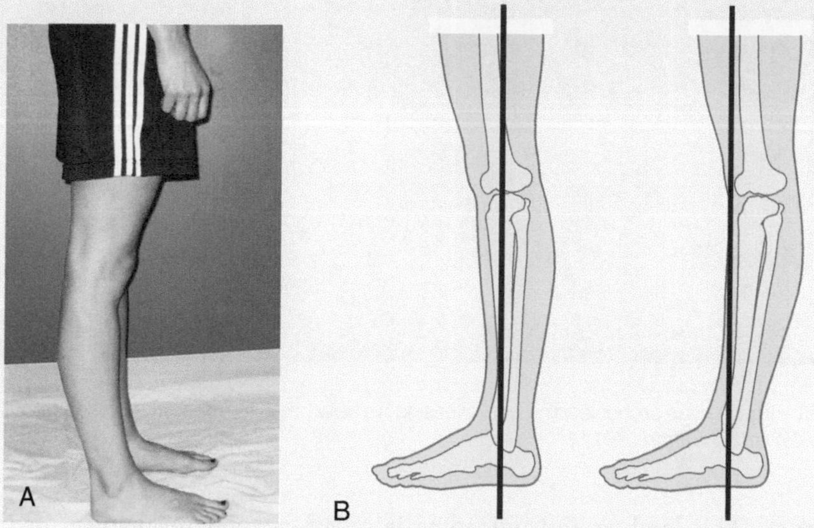

Fig. 3.21 (A) Over extended knees are a typical feature in the hypermobile tissue. (B) Connective tissue is hyperelastic causing hypermobile movement of joints.

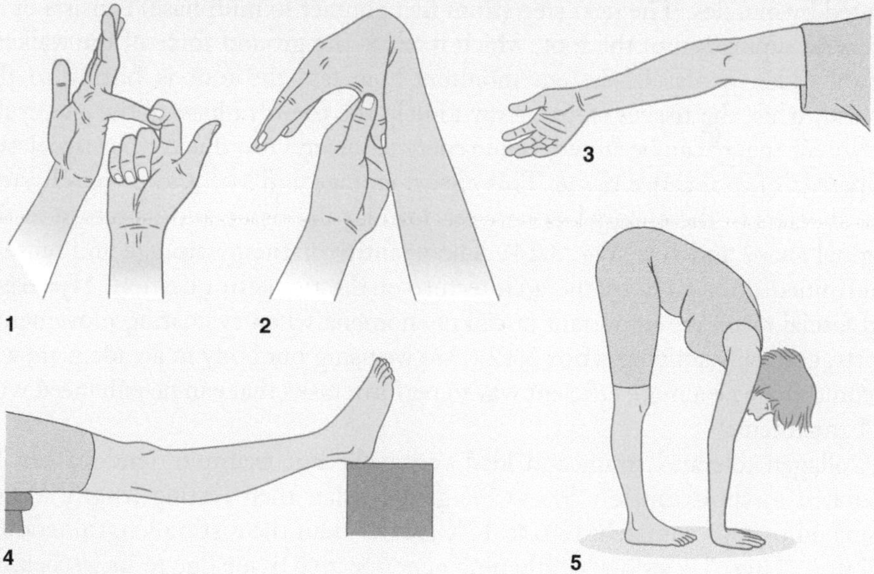

Fig. 3.22 Beighton's scoring is used as an assessment tool for hypermobility. *(From Kenyon (2009).)*

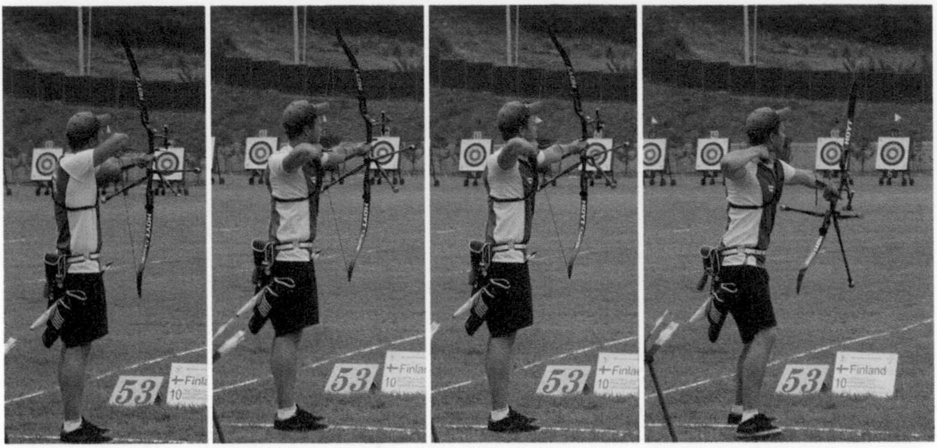

Fig. 3.23 Image of an archer loading and releasing his bow helps to understand fascial recoil in the tissue. *(From Sahrmann, 2011.)*

efficiency. This loading and unloading is called catapult mechanism or fascial recoil (Chaitow, 2014; Schleip and Müller, 2012). Loading is like the archer flexing a bow and then releasing the energy when the arrow is shot (Fig. 3.23). A simple example of fascial recoil is walking. The first step is a push created by muscles. The next step (from first contact to midphase) consists of an eccentric supination of the foot, which receives the ground force of the walker's weight. The myofascial system monitors how fast the foot is hitting to the ground, while the tissues store energy to help the toe-off phase of the gait cycle.

Not all energy can be stored. Some energy is always lost due to the viscoelastic properties of connective tissue. This energy storage and loss is known as hysteresis. It refers to the energy lost between loading the tissue and its return to the original shape and size (Fig. 3.24). The quantity of energy storage and reuse is determined principally by the architecture of the tissue in question. Hysteresis and fascial recoil are important fascial phenomena when evaluating movements, sports, and daily activities (Box 3.12). Are we using our body in an adequate way or could there be a more efficient way to perform tasks that can be enhanced with FM treatment?

Collagen tolerates strain and load very well. For example, tendons can be stretched to approximately 5% to 8% greater than their resting length. When stretched to approximately 10% to 12% greater than the resting length, tendons will tear. "Creep" is a slow lengthening of connective tissue due to its viscoelastic properties. Creep will happen over weeks, months, or years as opposed to one stretching event or exercise or even treatment intervention. A person who habitually stands in a hyperlordotic posture (forward tilted pelvis and lumbar spine lordosis) may be at risk for low back pain (Sorensen et al., 2015). Prolonged

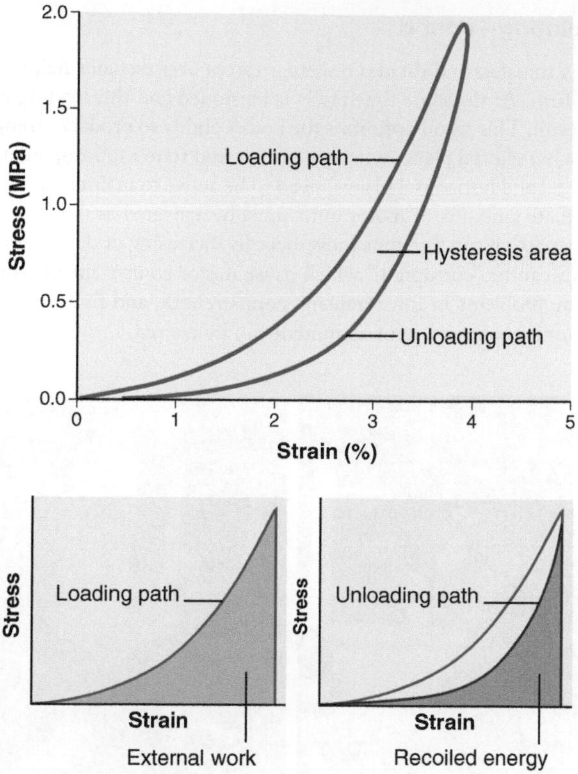

Fig. 3.24 Hysteresis. *(From Stecco, 2013.)*

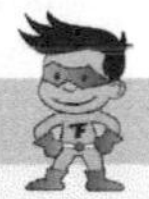

BOX 3.12 Squatting

Squatting (Fig. 3.25) has an interesting relationship to fascia. It is normally used in strength training in modern societies. In past centuries humans have used the squat as a normal routine. Many jobs, works, or chores have been carried out in squatting position, as in childbirth. The squat is a combination of joint movement, fascial gliding, fascial recoil, and muscular strength. It requires our body to be controlled, elastic, and strong. A squat begins in a standing position. To stand stabile we require individual joint awareness. This happens with help of the mechanoreceptors in joint capsules, ligaments, muscles, and fascia. They all send signals to the sensory cortex of the central nervous system (CNS). In that system we have a representation of the "input" information. With this information our CNS switches on the required motor units. If there is an extra weight or other resistance, more units are needed to maintain the same posture.

As the squat movement occurs the motor cortex sends signals ("output") to the motor units allowing the centre of gravity of the body to shift down and backwards and downward in the sagittal plane. The lumbar area is maintaining a neutral position by way of the back and abdominal muscles, while the legs and pelvic muscles work eccentrically controlling the

Continued

BOX 3.12 Squatting—cont'd

movement. Fascia transfers and divides muscular forces over distance helping the body to be more steady and firm. At the same time fascia is tensioned and this loading of forces releases later as a fascial recoil. This recoil optimizes the body's ability to produce strength using stored energy. The squat is a sagittal plane movement (ante- and retro motion), but at the same time, other planes (frontal and horizontal planes) need to be active to maintain a smooth and steady movement. Adequate amounts of motor units must be activated as the CNS controls movement and when needed, it can fine tune movement by increasing or decreasing strength levels. Input to the CNS can be "corrupted," which cause motor control misinterpretations. These errors can generate problems in force transmission, strength, and fine-tuning. In these cases movements are not smooth and joint alignment can be altered.

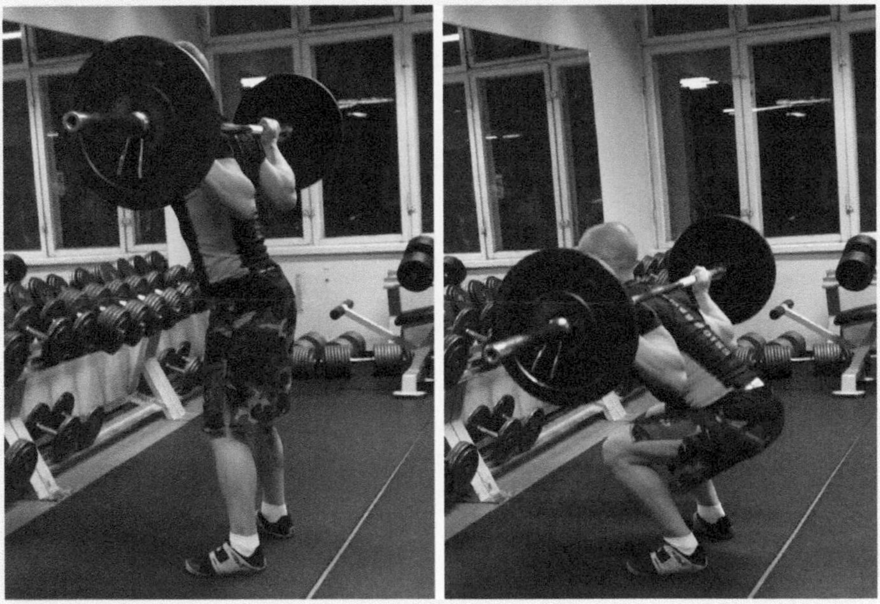

Fig. 3.25 Squatting is a combination of coordination, mobility, strength, fascial gliding and recoil.

hyperlordotic posture will load connective tissue in the lumbar and pelvic area. Collagen will adapt to this position and will be repeatedly loaded and lengthened. Such bad habits, repeated over and over again during days, months, and years, will result in creep and eventually pain (Fig. 3.26).

Fascia is a key element that binds different tissues together. It also transfers forces created by muscle cells to the neighbouring tissues and over distances. Fascial tissue is like a bridge transferring and sharing the forces. Pihlman et al. (2015) and Yousefi et al. (2013) have determined that fascial connections are able to

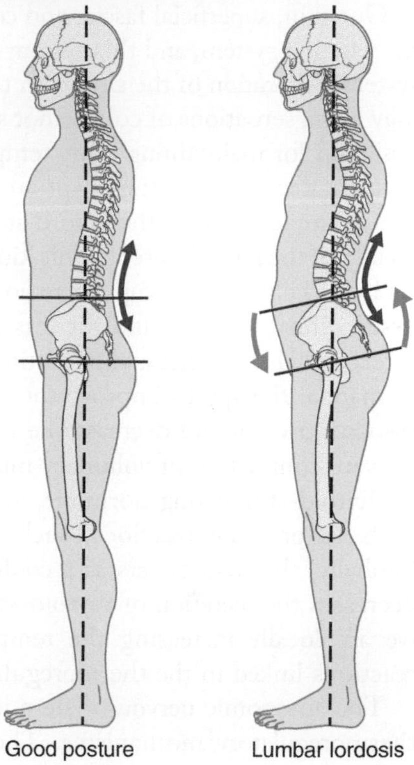

Fig. 3.26 Hyperlordotic posture is typical misalignment of the body, where proprioception and coordination is altered. *(From Kenyon and Kenyon, 2009.)*

increase muscular force. Increased strength enables bigger lever arms and/or pulley-like actions. If connective tissue has the ability to increase strength, then it should be able to tolerate and store forces.

Fascia and Thermoregulation

Environmental and climatic stress is related to our body via skin and superficial fascia. Overall, our bodies compensate very well to prevailing temperatures and conditions. People who are used to living in cold climates have trouble regulating their body when travelling to the south or *vice versa*. It may take time to adapt our bodies to a new environment. When our thermoregulatory system is working appropriately the adaptation will happen smoothly. Inside the hypodermis and superficial fascia we find all the receptors for temperature. Besides, the superficial fascia and the retinacula cutis help to maintain storage of the fat tissue. The brown fat is usually present inside the superficial fascia. Finally, the superficial fascia envelops the superficial vascular plexus that is fundamental for thermoregulation. We can imagine that an alteration of the superficial fascia and skin ligaments will affect thermoregulation. One example of this alteration is cellulitis.

Our skin, superficial fascia, and connective tissue have close connections with the vascular system, and this system is tightly connected to the thermoregulatory system. Alteration of the shunts in the arteriovenous framework including fascia may cause sensations of cold or hot skin. Thermoregulatory systems are not only designed for maintaining body temperature but also participate in its functions that are necessary for the adaption to environmental changes inside our body. For example Inuits gather more storage fat than people in the south and the quality of the fat is different. This kind of brown adipose tissue can be found especially in the neck and scapular regions. It is easier to expose this kind of adipose tissue directly to heat and for this reason it is important for thermoregulation (Stecco, 2015). In therapeutic settings local application of cold and heat are used in manual therapy to improve the effects of treatment. Locally, cold will cause vasoconstriction and decrease the temperature of the tissue. Globally, cold can activate contraction of voluntary muscles and may lead to increase of secretions of thyroid-stimulating hormone, adrenaline, and other hormones. Heat locally leads to opposite reactions, such as vasodilation and sweating of the skin. Globally, this system acts as a cooling system for our body. Heat also globally decreases the secretion of thyroid-stimulating hormone. By manipulating fascia we are locally increasing the temperature of the tissue and activating these reactions linked to the thermoregulatory system.

The autonomic nervous system under control of the hypothalamus regulates thermoregulatory mechanisms. The thermogenic centre of the hypothalamus and its neurons trigger mechanisms related to heat production. Fever is one example of stress reactions of the thermoregulatory system. Tissue damage or infection may shift the temperature of the body to a fever state. Fever is a contraindication for FM treatment. On the other hand, indications for treatment would include painful cellulitis or sensations of a cold feeling in some areas. Thermoregulatory problems can provoke sensations of warmth or cold in the specific areas of superficial fascia known as quadrants in FM (Fig. 3.27) (Stecco and Stecco, 2014).

Fascia as a Part of the Immune System

The immune system includes important processes allowing our body to identify antigens, viruses, and bacteria. This system represents the fortress of our body. Our first line of defence is the skin that protects us from environmental stress factors, such as pollution, heat, cold, or topical creams. The lymphatic system is our second line of defence and the third line of defence includes tonsils, thymus, spleen, deep lymph nodes, and autonomic ganglias. Superficial fascia can be visualized as a military trench where our own soldiers are hidden. Stressors coming from the outside or inside of our body are trying to attack our fortress. Pollution, food, and mental and physical stress are examples of factors that are compromising our immunologic system. To learn more about fascial connections and deeper

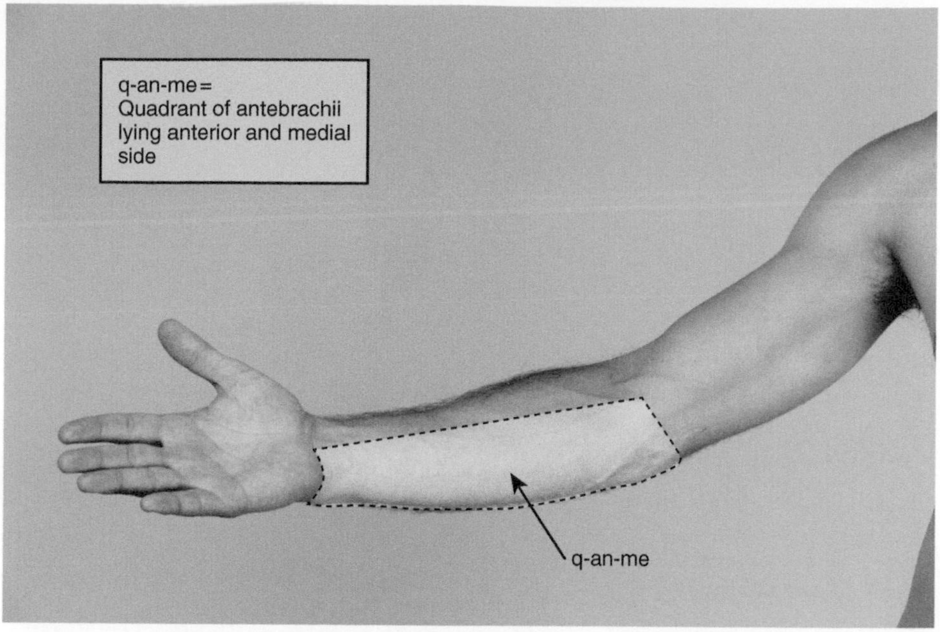

Fig. 3.27 Example of ante-medial quadrant of the forearm.

understanding of the immunologic system, read *Fascial Manipulation for Internal Dysfunctions* by Luigi and Carla Stecco (Stecco and Stecco, 2014) (Fig. 3.28).

FM utilizes a more superficial and lighter manipulation on affected quadrants when treating from an immunologic point of view (FM Part III course). FM practitioners will treat the most densified points to modify the ground substance toward normal fluidity. Conditions like fibromyalgia and acute rheumatoid arthritis may benefit from this approach, especially in the early stages of these conditions. Every part of our body is connected and every function of our body is integrated to allow normal functioning of cells, tissues, muscles, and organs. FM attempts to balance the body and help it to maintain homeostasis. Dysfunction and misaligned posture might predispose us to abnormal tension and stress in our connective tissue system affecting to the whole system.

Classic ideas of mechanics are important, but we advance our knowledge by opening our minds to allow new concepts as we study the living tissue. Also, from fresh cadavers we can continue to improve our knowledge of anatomy and histology. We can eventually learn how to truly map the human body. Using ultrasound, elastography, MRI, and other modalities to investigate the living body helps us learn even more about the function and connections in our body from the fascial point of view.

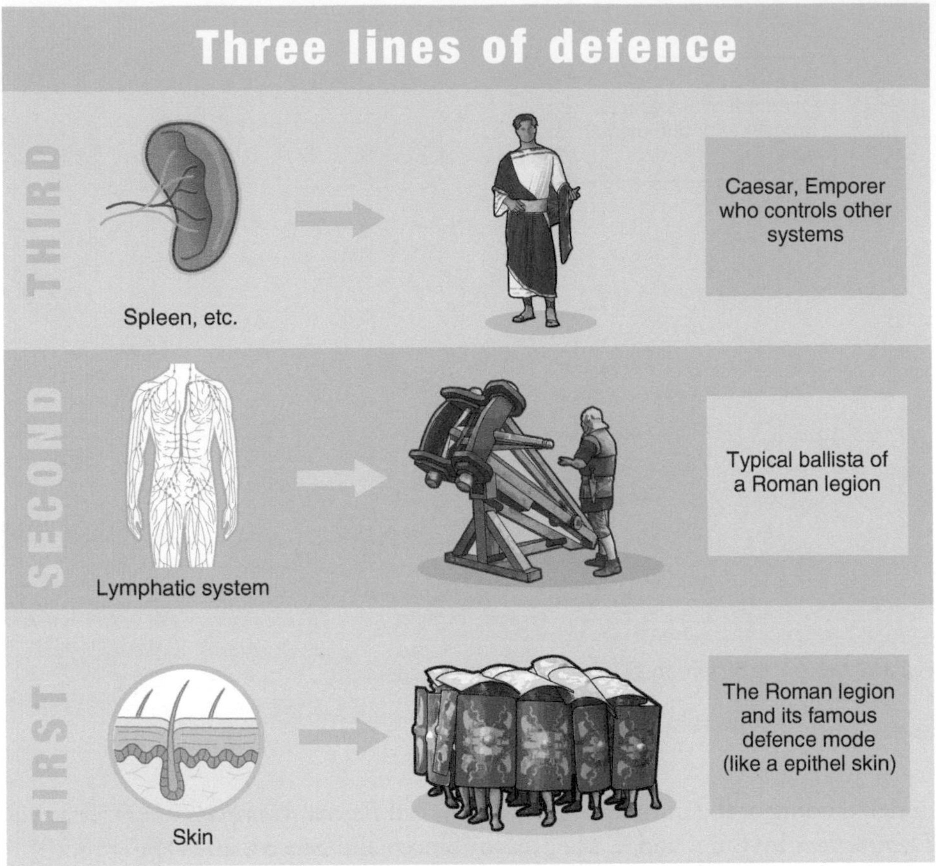

Fig. 3.28 Three defence lines of the body – our immunological defence viewed as a Roman army.

References

Adler, S., Beckers, D., Buck, M., 2008. PNF in Practice, third ed. Heidelberg, Springer-Verlag, Berlin.

Bednar, D., William, F., Simon, G., 1995. Observations on the pathomorphology of the thoracolumbar fascia in chronic mechanical back pain: a microscopic study. Spine. Vol. 20, Issue 10.

Benjamin, M., 2009. The fascia of the limbs and back — review. J. Anat. 214, 1–18.

Chaitow, L. (editor), 2014. Fascial Dysfunction, manual therapy approaches. Handspring Publishing.

Chiarugi, G., Bucciante, L., 1975. Istituzioni di Anatomia dell'uomo, 11th ed. Vallardi-Piccin, Padova. First edition 1904.

Cruz-Montecinos, C., González Blanche, A., López Sánchez, D., Cerda, M., Sanzana-Cuche, R., Cuesta-Vargas, A., 2015. In vivo relationship between pelvis motion and deep fascia displacement of the medial gastrocnemius: anatomical and functional implications. J. Anat. http://dx.doi.org/10.1111/joa.12370.

De Luca, C.J., Mambrito, B., 1987. Voluntary control of motor units in human antagonist muscles: coactivation and reciprocal activation. J. Neurophysiol. 58, 3.

Deising, S., Weinkauf, B., Blunk, J., Obreja, O., Schmelz, M., Rukwied, R., 2012. NGF-evoked sensitization of muscle fascia nociceptors in humans. J. Pain. 153 (8), 1673–1679. http://dx.doi.org/10.1016/j.pain.2012.04.033.

Findley, T., Chaudry, H., Dhar, S., 2015. Transmission of muscle force to fascia during exercise. J. Bodyw. Mov. Ther. 19 (1), 119–123. http://dx.doi.org/10.1016/j.jbmt.2014.08.010. Epub 2014 Sep 3.

Fukunaga, T., Kawakami, Y., Kubo, K., Kanehisa, H., 2002. Muscle and tendon interaction during human movement. Exerc. Sport Sci. Rev. 30 (3), 106–110.

Gracovetsky, S., 2007. First Fascia Research Congress, Boston, MA.

Grahame, R., 2000. The revised (Brighton 1998) criteria for the diagnosis of benign joint hypermobility syndrome (BJHS). J. Rheumatol. 27, 1777–1779.

Huijing, P.A., 1999. Muscle as a collagen fiber reinforced composite: a review of force transmission in muscle and whole limb. J. Biomech 32 (4), 329–345.

Huijing, P.A., Baan, G.C., 2008. Myofascial force transmission via extramuscular pathways occurs between antagonistic muscles. Cells Tissues Organs 188, 400–414.

Jensen, M.C., Brant-Zawadski, M.N., Obuchowski, N., et al., 1994. Magnetic resonance imaging of the lumbar spine in people without back pain. N. Engl. J. Med. 331 (2), 69–73.

Kenyon, K., Kenyon, J., 2009. The Physiotherapist's Pocket Book. Churchill Livingstone.

Ker, R., 1999. The design of soft collagenous load-bearing tissues. J. Exp. Biol. 202, 3315–3324.

Langevin, H., 2006. Connective tissue: A body-wide signaling network? Medical hypothesis. Elsevier Vol. 66, Issue 6, pp. 1074–1077. http://dx.doi.org/10.1016/j.mehy.2005.12.032.

Langevin, H., Fox, J.R., Koptiuch, C., Badger, G.J., Greenan-Naumann, A.C., Bouffard, N.A., et al., 2011. Reduced thoracolumbar fascia shear strain in human chronic low back pain. BMC Musculoskelet. Disord. 12, 203.

Levin, S.M., 2006. Tensegrity: The new biomechanics. In: Hutson, M., Ellis, R. (Eds.), Textbook of musculoskeletal medicine. Oxford University Press.

Luomala, T., Pihlman, M., Stecco, C., 2015. Comparison of the equine and human fascial system. Fascia Research Congress IV Book. Elsevier, Washington.

Maganaris, C., Paul, J., 1999. In vivo human tendon mechanical properties. J. Physiol. 521, 307–331.

Marchuk, C., Stecco, C., 2015. The role of connective tissue in the embryology of the musculoskeletal system: towards a paradigm shift. F1000 Res. http://dx.doi.org/10.12688/F1000research.6824.1.

Panjabi, M.M., 1992. The stabilizing system of the spine. Part I. Function, dysfunction, adaptation, and enhancement. J. Spinal Disord. 5 (4), 383–389. discussion 397.

Panjabi, M.M., 2006. A hypothesis of chronic back pain: ligament subfailure injuries lead to muscle control dysfunction. Eur. Spine J. 15 (5), 668–676. Epub 2005 Jul 27.

Patel, T., Lieber, R., 1997. Force transmission in skeletal muscle: from actomyosin to external tendons. Exerc. Sport Sci. Rev. http://dx.doi.org/10.1249/00003677-199700250-00014.

Pihlman, M., Luomala, T., Heiskanen, J., Stecco, C., 2015. Anatomical findings and co-operative function of m. deltoid and m. brachialis. Fascia Research Congress IV Book. Elsevier, Washington.

Purslow, P., 2010. Muscle fascia and force transmission. J. Bodyw. Mov. Ther. 4, 411–417. http://dx.doi.org/10.1016/j.jbmt.2010.01.005.

Roman, M., Chaudhry, H., Bukiet, B., Stecco, A., Findley, T.W., 2013. Mathematical analysis of the flow of hyaluronic acid around fascia during manual therapy motions. J. Am. Osteopath. Assoc. http://dx.doi.org/10.7556/jaoa.2013.021.

Rosso, C., Schuetz, P., Polzer, C., Weisskopf, L., Studler, U., Valderrabano, V., 2012. Physiological achilles tendon length and its relation to tibia length. Clin. J. Sport Med. http://dx.doi.org/10.1097/JSM.0b013e3182639a3e.

Sahrmann, S., 2011. Movement System Impairment Syndromes of the Extremities, Cervical and Thoracic Spines. Mosby.

Sanchis-Alfonso, V., Rosello-Sastre, E., 2000. Immunohistochemical analysis for neural markers of the lateral retinaculum in patients with isolated symptomatic patellofemoral malalignment. A neuroanatomic basis for anterior knee pain in the active young patient. Am. J. Sports Med. 28 (5), 725–731.

Scarr G. 2014. Biotensegrity, the structural basis of life. Handspring Publishing.

Schilder, A., Hoheisel, U., Magerl, W., Benrath, J., Klein, T., Treede, R.D., 2014. Deep tissue and back pain: stimulation of the thoracolumbar fascia with hypertonic saline. Schmerz. http://dx.doi.org/10.1007/s00482-013-1373-3.

Schleip, R., 2003. Fascial plasticity — a new neurobiological explanation. J. Bodyw. Mov. Ther. 7 (1), 11–19 and 7 (2), 104–116.

Schleip, R., Müller, D., 2012. Training principals for fascial connective tissue: scientific foundation and suggested practical application. J. Bodyw. Mov. Ther. http://dx.doi.org/10.1016/j.jbmt.2012.06.007.

Schleip, R., Müller, D., 2013. Training principles for fascial connective tissues: scientific foundation and suggested practical applications. J. Bodyw. Mov. Ther. 17, 103–115.

Shumway-Cook, A., Woollacott, M.H., 2007. Motor Control — Translating Research to Clinical Practice, third ed. Lippincott Williams and Wilkins.

Sorensen, C., Norton, B., Callaghan, J., Hwang, C., Van Dillen, L., 2015. Is lumbar lordosis related to low back pain development during prolonged standing? Man. Ther. http://dx.doi.org/10.1016/j.math.2015.01.001.

Standring, S., 2008. Gray's Anatomy: The anatomical basic of clinical practice. 40th edition. Churchill Livingstone, Elsevier. First published: Parker & Son 1858.

Stecco, C., 2015. Functional Atlas of the Human Fascial System. Churchill Livingstone, Elsevier.

Stecco, C., Gagey, O., Belloni, A., et al., 2007. Anatomy of the deep fascia of the upper limb. Second part: study of innervation. Morphologie 91, 38–43.

Stecco, L., Stecco, C., 2009. Fascial Manipulation Practical Part. Piccin, Padua, Italy.

Stecco, L., Stecco, C., 2014. Fascial Manipulation for Internal Dysfunction. Piccin, Padua, Italy.

Stecco, A., Wolfgang, G., Robert, H., Fullerton, B., Stecco, C., 2013. The anatomical and functional relation between gluteus maximus and fascia lata. J. Bodyw. Mov. Ther. 17, 512–517.

Stecco, A., Meneghini, A., Stern, R., Stecco, C., Imamura, M., 2014. Ultrasonography in myofascial neck pain: randomized clinical trial for diagnosis and follow-up. Surg. Radiol. Anat. 36, 243–253.

Tezars, J., Hoheisel, U., Wiedenhöfer, B., Mense, S. 2011. Sensory innervation of the thoracolumbar fascia in rats and humans. Neuroscience 194, 302–308.

Tortora, G., Derrickson, B., 2011. Principles of Anatomy and Physiology, Organization, Support and Movement, and Control Systems of the Human Body, 13th ed. John Wiley and Sons.

Vleeming, A., Pool-Goudzwaard, A., Stoeckart, R., van Wingerden, J.-P., Snijders, C., 1995. The Posterior Layer of the Thoracolumbar Fascia. Its Function in Load Transfer From Spine to Legs. Spine. Vol. 20, Issue 7.

Wilke, J., Engeroff, T., Nürberger, F., Vogt, L., Banzer, W., 2015. Anatomical study of the morphological continuity between iliotibial tract and the fibularis longus fascia. Surg. Radiol. Anat. http://dx.doi.org/10.1007/s00276-015-1585-6.

Yousefi, H., Baniasadi, M., Rostami, M., 2013. The role of fascia around the patellar tendon in force transmission: an experimental study on sheep stifle joint. Biomed. Eng. Res. 2, 71–78.

CHAPTER 4

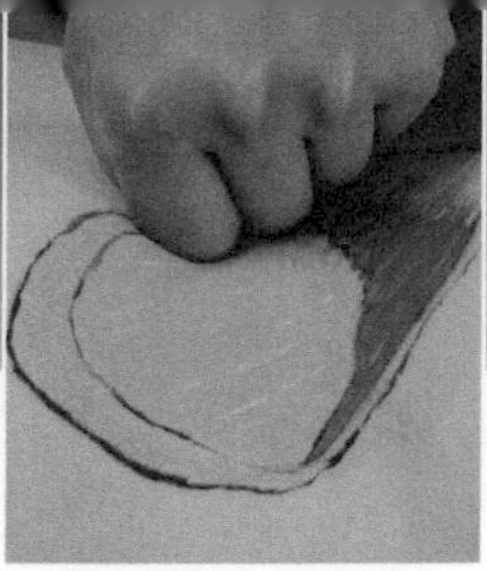

Fascial Manipulation

People have been suffering with musculoskeletal problems from the beginning of time, usually due to overwork, injury, stress, or inactivity. Problems are often described as occurring for no apparent reason. Early texts about treatment methods originated in China in the age of the Yellow Emperor, Huangdi Neijing. *The Emperor's Inner Canon*, his famous text, was translated 2000 years later into French and this led later to the development of classic massage, where Greco-Roman traditions were incorporated into Eastern traditions. Previously, the Sumerians and Egyptians had cuneiform scripts and hieroglyphs about treatment methods. Over the decades new treatment methods have continued to develop all over the world. Even today, many new healing methods have drawn information from previous healing systems such as acupuncture and its related meridians. Nowadays, due to computers and new methods of manufacturing, people are more sedentary than ever. In the light of history we have turned from hunter-gatherers to passive sitters and standers (Fig. 4.1). It is estimated that 85% of the public suffers at one time or another with what is known as myofascial pain syndrome. According to fascial manipulation (FM), altered fascia is the key element responsible for this syndrome (see Video 9).

With so many methods of treatment available, one may ask, why FM? FM is one of the few methods that evaluate patients from a global point of view. Based on current research and clinical experience, the myofascial kinetic chain can finally be realized. That is why in FM, the history of the patient is so important. For instance, a 10-year-old ankle sprain can often be the cause of a chronic back complaint. FM, by way of the anatomy and physiology of the fascial system, reveals a direct connection along fascial planes that are responsible for "connecting" the whole body. The location of pain is often misleading with regard to causation. The case history of an old trauma or injury even dating back to childhood becomes relevant. Every patient is recognized as an individual and rarely are patients with the same complaint treated the same way. FM attempts to create homeostasis to allow the body to heal itself. Human desires are still the same: we want to be pain free and able to do our daily tasks with ease. This is a method that combines knowledge with physical sensitivity. The final decision as to how and where a patient will be treated is based on their case history, movement, palpatory verification and clinical reasoning.

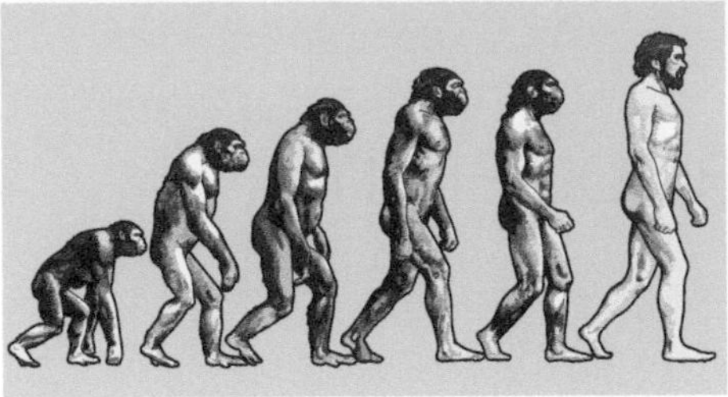

Fig. 4.1 Human evolution.

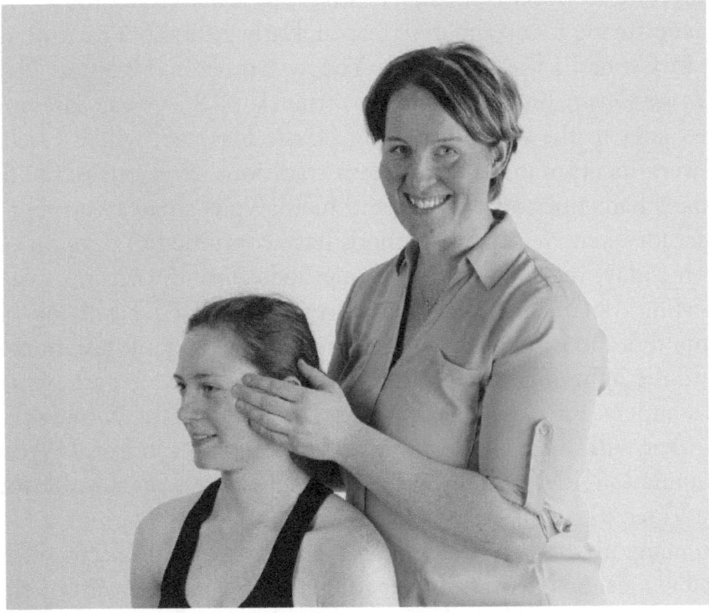

Fig. 4.2 Fascial manipulation is a lifelong learning process.

Presently, FM is taught in three levels. Level I is for the basic understanding of the anatomy and physiology of fascia, the centres of coordination (CCs), and its sequences. Level II concentrates on the centres of fusion via diagonals and spirals. Level III helps us solve internal dysfunction by evaluating the CCs and centres of fusion (CFs) of the body's total tensile structure as it relates to the fascia of internal organs. Master classes are also available for practitioners who have completed the courses and desire to continue to improve their skills. Many FM practitioners belong to local study groups who share their experiences. FM seeks the truth and its methods are always improving with ongoing research. After you have mastered the basics, you will begin to appreciate the significant healing power of FM (Fig. 4.2).

Treatment of the fascia is important from many aspects. Nowadays, new studies confirm the idea that fascia is a principal source of pain, and is responsible for normal proprioception and muscle force transmission. Imagine if everything was removed from our body except the fascial tissue, we would see a three-dimensional outline of our body. Evolution has created this tissue to "provide a structural framework for the body and maintain the anatomic form of the organs and systems, to cushion and protect surrounding organs and tissues, to aid in metabolism whereby blood and waste metabolites can pass through, store energy and regulate the diffusion of substances" (Stecco, 2015). Fascia participates in numerous bodily functions. Some of those functions still wait to be revealed. FM expands our knowledge concerning myofascial dysfunction and disorders by the recent revelation that it is a sensory organ. It also helps us to understand more complex disorders related to internal dysfunction.

Main Principles

To help understand the practical use of FM, it is necessary to first comprehend its underlying principles (Box 4.1). This chapter will discuss the biomechanical model of FM, including segments, myofascial units (MFUs), CCs, centres of perception (CPs), and related sequences. The locations of some of the CCs are listed to help understand the FM concept for treatment of the myofascial system. CFs, diagonals, and spirals are introduced from the functional point of view. This book is not intended to be used as a treatment manual.

BOX 4.1 The FM Method in a Nutshell

In the fascial manipulation (FM) method we can locate specific points called centres of coordination (CCs) and centres of fusions (CFs). They represent the tensional network of our body, the treatment matrix. The idea of segments (eg, neck, shoulder, or knee) specifies the localization of these points. CCs can be found in areas where muscle forces meet and they can be categorized into sequences (series of CC points between segments). CFs are classified into diagonals and spirals and they are located closer to joints and retinacula. The whole list of CCs and CFs can be found in the *Fascial Manipulation Practical Part* (Stecco and Stecco, 2009) and upcoming books.

The FM system includes case history, movement verification, palpatory verification, treatment, and reassessment. The main goal of FM is to balance the body to allow painless function. From the case history the hypothesis is decided upon to determine which segments may require treatment. After the case history and movement and palpatory verification, treatment is performed with fingers, knuckles, or elbows on predetermined points. It is always necessary that in each visit points are treated that result in a balancing of agonists and antagonists of a sequence. Reassessment of impaired function (muscle tests, etc.) is used to evaluate the effects of a treatment session during the treatment to ensure that you are treating the correct sequence and at the conclusion of the treatment to confirm that there is maximum improvement. Specific FM assessment charts are used to collect data and record results (Fig. 4.3).

Continued

BOX 4.1 ■ **The FM Method in a Nutshell—cont'd**

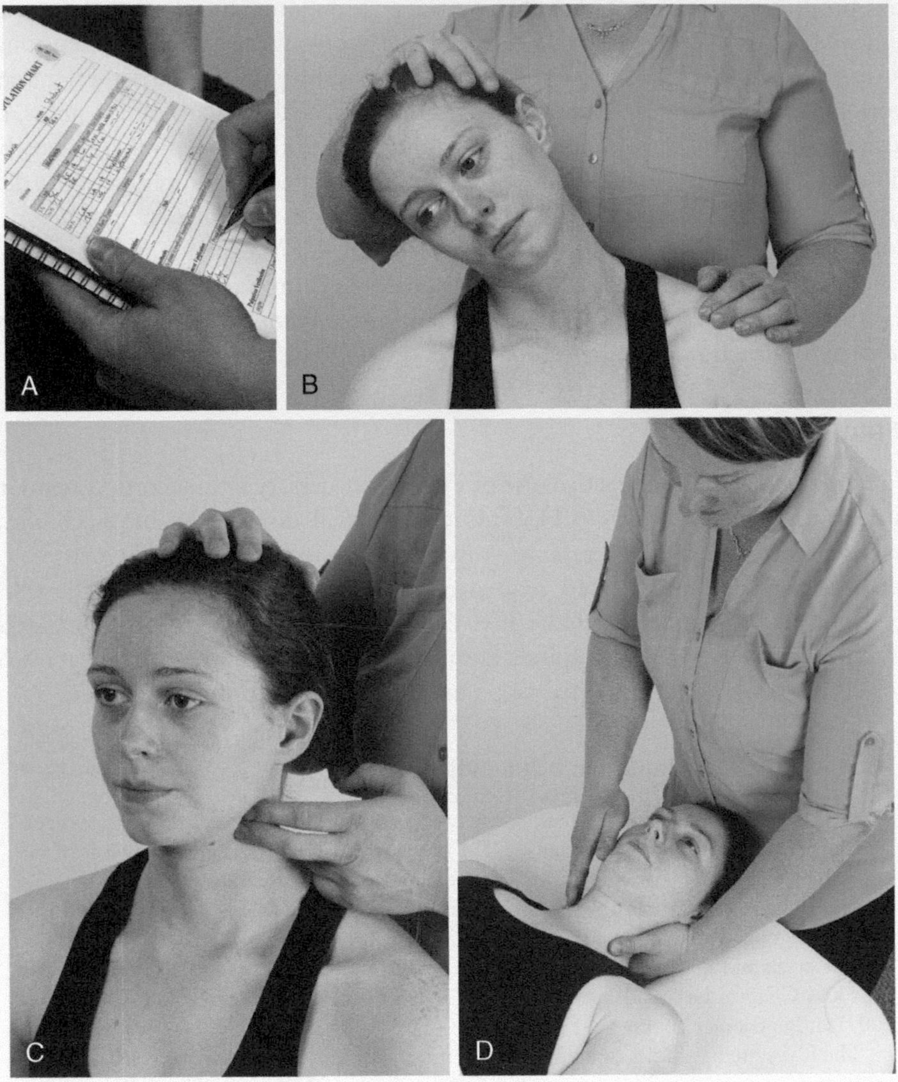

Fig. 4.3 The fascial manipulation method in a nutshell: case history, movement and palpatory verification, treatment, and reassessment.

Terminology

Luigi Stecco invented terminology and abbreviations for FM based on Latin. Using this universal language allows practitioners to communicate with other FM practitioners worldwide.

SEGMENTS

FM divides our body into 14 segments. One of the segments, the head (CP, caput), includes three subunits (points) recorded as CP1, CP2, and CP3. Each segment of a body represents a particular part of the body that is tested by movement verification and palpation verification to determine which segments require treatment. FM is almost always used on related segments either near each other or at a distance. For example, treatment of chronic lumbar pain may begin with treatment of leg points that are on a similar sequence of fascial points found in the lumbar area. The idea of segments is based on anatomy and functionality. Dividing body parts into segments (Fig. 4.4) helps to locate the causative and compensatory locations within the myofascial sequence.

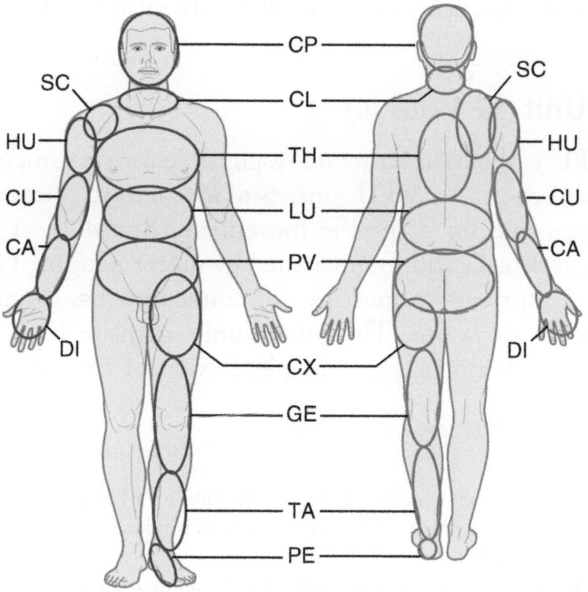

Fig. 4.4 Chart of segments. *CP*, caput, head, and three subunits (CP1, eyes; CP2, mandible; and CP3, ears); *CL*, collum, neck, C1–C7; *TH*, thorax, rib cage, and 12 thoracic vertebrae; *LU*, lumbar, lumbar vertebrae, and abdomen above the umbilicus to beneath xiphoid process; *PV*, pelvis, crest of ilium, sacrum, pubic symphysis, part of ischium; *CX*, coxa, hip joint, proximal half of thigh, sacrotuberous and sacrospinous ligaments; *GE*, genu, half of anterior thigh to tibial tuberosity, posteriorly to proximal one-third of triceps surae; *TA*, talus, myofascia beneath knee to proximal foot that moves the talus in three spatial planes; *PE*, pes, foot, part of calcaneus, tarsus, and all of metatarsal and phalangeal bones; *SC*, scapula, bones, and muscles of shoulder girdle; *HU*, humerus, GH joint, and fibre of deltoid, biceps brachii, triceps; *CU*, cupitus, distal two-thirds of upper arm, proximal one-third of forearm, biceps, brachioradialis, triceps; *CA*, Carpus, distal two-thirds of forearm, proximal row of carpals; *DI*, digiti, hand, distal carpals, metacarpals, and phalanges.

MOTOR DIRECTION TERMINOLOGY

Our brain thinks in general motor spatial directions and the final task. It does not interpret the function of individual muscles. The central nervous system (CNS) learns and adapts by creating motor programs. Motor programs are patterns of activation of sets of motor units. Luigi Stecco introduced a more functional language in FM based on motor direction.

Antemotion/antepulsion (AN) means that our body parts are moving forward in the sagittal plane. **Retromotion/retropulsion (RE)** represents backward movement in the sagittal plane. **Lateromotion/lateropulsion (LA)** refers to the frontal plane: side-bending or abduction of our body. **Mediomotion/mediopulsion (ME)** also refers to the frontal plane. In the upper and lower extremities it corresponds to the adduction. In the trunk it has an essentially perceptive role rather than indicating a specific movement. **Extrarotation (ER)** represents external rotation, a lateral outer motion in the horizontal plane. **Intrarotation (IR)** refers to inner, medial, or intrarotation movement in the horizontal plane. Sequences using these directions are introduced more closely later in the text.

Myofascial Unit (see Video 10)

In FM, the MFU is the basic structure responsible for movement of a segment in a particular direction. An MFU consists of motor units, nerves, veins, joints, and fascia responsible for a specific movement (Box 4.2). A motor unit is composed of muscle cells (fibre) innervated by motor neuron. The veins transport oxygen and nutrients to muscles and connective tissue and also act as a conduit for metabolic waste. The motor units activate both monoarticular and biarticular muscle fibres. For example, flexion of the elbow requires both

BOX 4.2

The myofascial unit (MFU) is considered a basic structure in FM (see Fig. 4.5). It is based on anatomical planes of movement and the body's ability to produce and control movements in specific directions. An MFU is:

1. Composed of a group of motor units that activate monoarticular and biarticular muscle fibres that move a body segment in a specific direction. A motor unit consists of a motor neuron and the multiple muscle fibres (cells) it innervates. Motor units activate muscle fibres that move one joint (monoarticular) and also muscles that cross over the joint (biarticular). For example, flexion of the elbow occurs when monoarticular (brachialis) and biarticular (biceps brachii) fibres are activated. Fibres are producing the movement in the same direction as in flexion of the elbow joint.
2. The joint that is moved.
3. The associated nerves (efferent, afferent, receptor [spindle cells], and vascular components).
4. The fascia that connects these elements together.

Continued

BOX 4.2 —cont'd

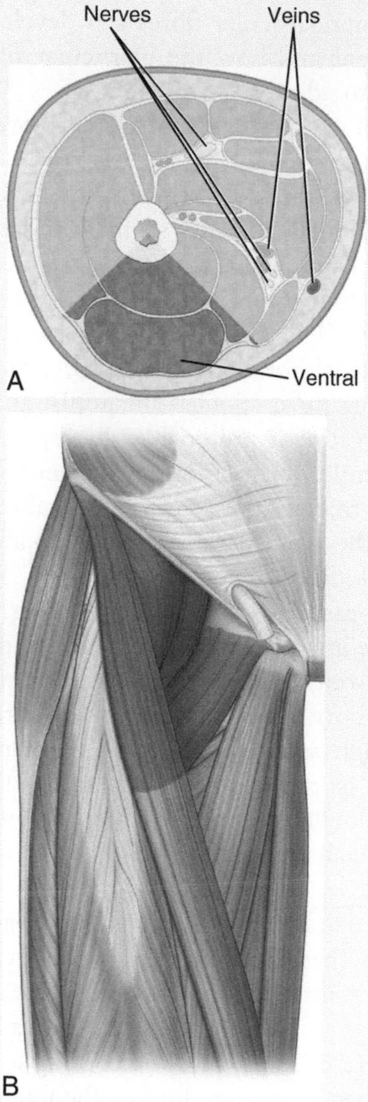

Fig. 4.5 (A) Cross-section of myofascial unit of AN-CX. (B) Anterior view of myofascial unit on AN-CX.

monoarticular (brachialis) and biarticular (biceps brachii) fibre activation. Fibres produce movement in the same direction like flexion of the elbow joint (forward—antemotion or antepulsion). Fascia is the element that unites these components together. If we analyse these muscular fibres, we can see how the monoarticular fibres are deeper than the biarticular ones, and how the mass of the monoarticular fibres is more voluminous than the mass of biarticular fibres. This explains why the monoarticular fibres can develop a higher quotient of strength during movement and how the biarticular fibres are more involved in transmitting tension to adjoining segments.

MFU names are based on anatomical planes of movement in specific directions. Every segment includes six myofascial units; two units for each of the three planes of movement. Movement of the segment can be identified in three planes (sagittal, frontal, and horizontal) and each segment in six directions, forward and backward (sagittal), lateral and medial (frontal), and internal or external rotation (horizontal). AN-HU means forward motion (agonist) and RE-HU means backward motion (antagonist). The same applies to lateral (LA-HU) and medial motion (ME-HU), external rotation (ER-HU), and internal rotation (IR-HU). These pairs are working as agonist–antagonist and this information is an important part of the treatment protocol with respect to creating balance in the segments. Consequently, for each joint, different vectors of movement in space are recognized. In treating these vectors it is always necessary to create a proper balance between the agonist and antagonist to allow proper coordination between the muscles and joints.

Segments and MFUs can be visualized by thinking about a cake (Fig. 4.6). Each piece of cake can be imagined as one direction of movement. You can take a piece of cake from the front (forward motion) or from the side (lateral motion). Also we can have a cake above the cake when we think of our body segments. The foot, ankle, knee, and thigh can be considered as segmental layers of the cake. In the limbs our cakes have six pieces per cake and in the trunk we have additional pieces (to be described below). By using terms like antemotion and retromotion, it is easier to understand which way our body parts are moving or which part of the cake is missing.

In each MFU described in FM, we find two separate areas: the first is the fascia covering the muscle belly that is considered the active component of the MFU. The second is around the joint and its components, that is the passive component that gets moved by muscle contraction. In the first area Stecco indicates a point, situated on the deep fascia, called the CC. According to FM theory, the force of the muscle fibres converges on these points, as the force of the horses converges on the coachman. The coordination of these tensile forces in the MFU is determined by the continuity of the fascia. Around the joint, finally, we find an area called the CP where the patient feels the pain.

Motor units and MFUs are terms we use when describing CCs and CFs. Areas of the MFU are the spaces where identifiable points, CCs and CFs, are formed by vectorial forces. In FM, lines of segments formed by CCs are called sequences. CFs along segments form diagonals and spirals. These lines and points are responsible of the coordination and refinement of myofascial movement.

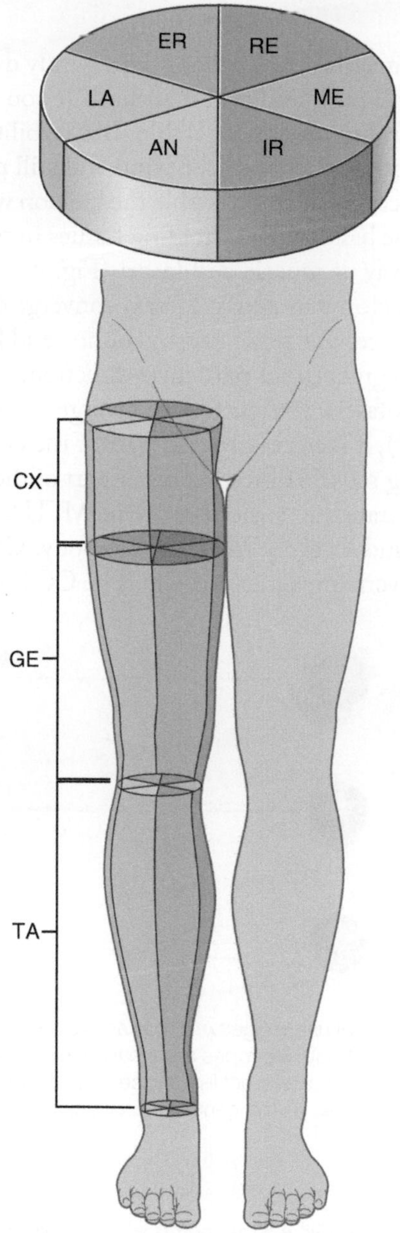

Fig. 4.6 Cake of segments.

CENTRES OF COORDINATION

CCs and fascia can be imagined as a balloon on a windy day. If you hold the balloon on a rope, wind will push and pull it around. If you take another rope and attach it to the balloon it becomes more stable. But stability occurs only between those two ropes. In all other directions the wind will still pull it. The more ropes you add from other directions the more stable the balloon will become. Fasciae act like ropes attached to the balloon, thus holding tissues in place helping to control and transfer forces by way of muscle and fascia (Fig. 4.7). The CC is the point where all these ropes (vectorial muscular forces) converge during muscle contraction (Box 4.3). These forces are generated by mono- and biarticular fibres of the MFU moving a body segment in a particular direction.

In order that this myofascial stretch/force converges onto a specific point of the fascia (what we call CC), it is necessary that part of the epimysial fascia is free to slide over the underlying muscle fibres. Another part of the fascia is inserted onto the bone in order to separate the tensioning of one MFU from the successive unit. This architecture is found in every MFU in the body. CCs are usually situated within the deep fascia overlying a muscle belly. The CC is rarely close to the joint.

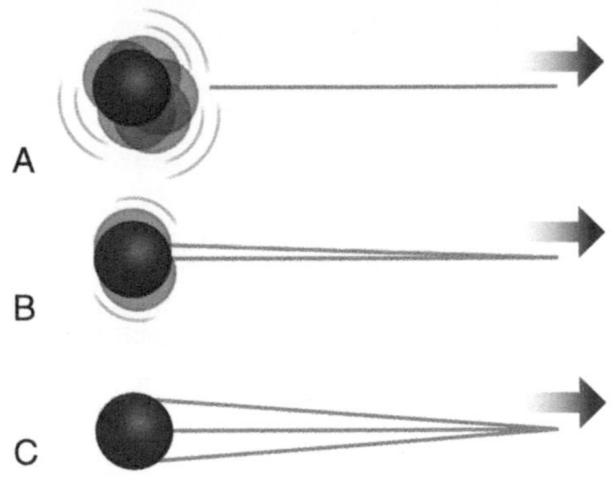

Fig. 4.7 Stability of the myofascial unit imaged with ball and ropes. (A) One rope is not enough to stabilize the movement of the ball. (B) Two ropes are creating more stability. Adding the third rope (C) will stabilize the ball even more. Fasciae act like a rope to hold tissues in place and control their movements. The ball can be imaged as the centre of coordination (CC).

BOX 4.3 ▪ CC

Centres of coordination (CCs) (Fig. 4.8) are points where the vectorial muscle forces meet in deep fascia. They act like a Roman chariot. If one of the horses is pulling too much, the driver has a hard time handling the chariot and the direction of the movement will change (Fig. 4.9). The CC can be seen as the driver of the chariot and the tensional lines represent the horses. If the driver (CC) is not able to handle the horses, the whole chariot will suffer, leading to dysfunction. Chariots join other chariots with their CCs to form a sequence as if they are a line of chariots in a parade. Every chariot (CC) has its own role and the proper alignment and connection of these chariots will create a pain-free movement pattern.

Continued

BOX 4.3 CC—cont'd

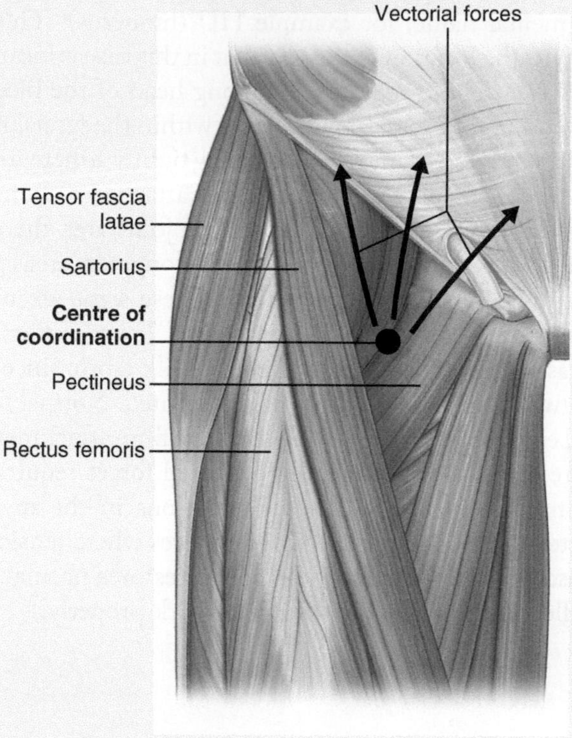

Fig. 4.8 Centre of coordination visualized with vectors.

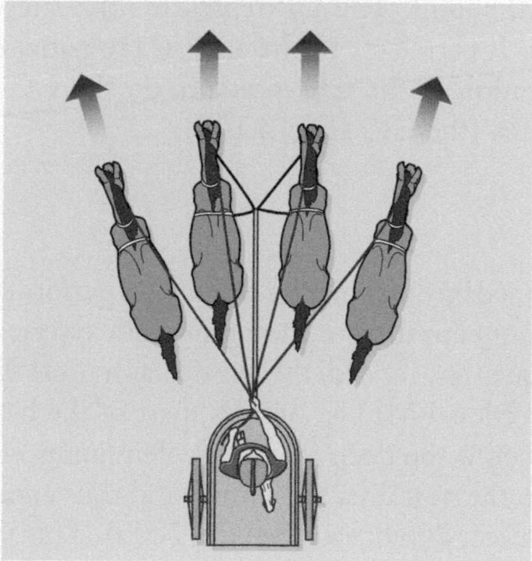

Fig. 4.9 Centre of coordination: metaphor of a Roman chariot.

Nomenclature of the points is created first by using the abbreviation of the direction of movement, for example AN (antemotion), and then adding the abbreviation of the segmental name, for example HU (humerus). This combination, AN-HU, represents the location of the CC that in this case is located on the anterior part of the upper deltoid medial to the long head of the biceps tendon.

Direction of movement occurs along vectors within the fascial net. Depending on the area, fascia may be freely movable or it may tightly adhere to the underlying or surrounding tissue, while in some places it is attached to bone. There is less movement of fascial layers near the joint. In the joint area there is more need for proprioception and stabilization. In broad elongated areas where muscles and fascia meet, more movement is required. These areas are mostly designed for force transmission and movement (upper and lower extremities). In these areas, layers of fascia can glide like two pieces of silk fabric since the loose connective tissue between these layers is normally hydrated. Normal fascial tension is created by fascial expansions of muscles and muscle fibre attachments. All of these characteristics are responsible for creating vectorial forces requiring normal CC and CF function. Dysfunctions and compensations in the myofascial system can alter the vectors inside the fascia. CCs are places where tension accumulates. Releasing the fascial dysfunction in these points restores normal muscle spindle function, thus allowing the nervous system to work properly.

CENTRES OF PERCEPTION

Every CC in the muscle has a referral area where perception occurs. If the unidirectional forces of the MFU are not synchronized an inappropriate or excessive tension will over stress the mechanoreceptors located in the capsule, ligaments, and tendons around the joint. The CP represents the site where movement at the joint is perceived. It correlates to the area where patients complain of pain. Because of a densification of the CC, pressure on the CC could cause referral of pain to the joint area (the CP) (Fig. 4.10).

SEQUENCES

The sequences are formed by the sum of all the MFUs performing movement in one direction. The precise organization of the aponeurotic fasciae gives the anatomical substratum for the sequences. Indeed, the biarticular muscle fibres composing each MFU connect unidirectional MFUs. Besides, part of the biarticular fibres found in each MFU inserts onto the deep fascia (myotendinous expansions) that links one joint (segment) to the next one, tensioning and thus connecting to other segments (Stecco and Stecco, 2009; Stecco et al., 2009). This myofascial continuity synchronizes the single MFU in order to develop forceful and precise movements. One myofascial sequence (MFS) synchronizes movement of several segments in

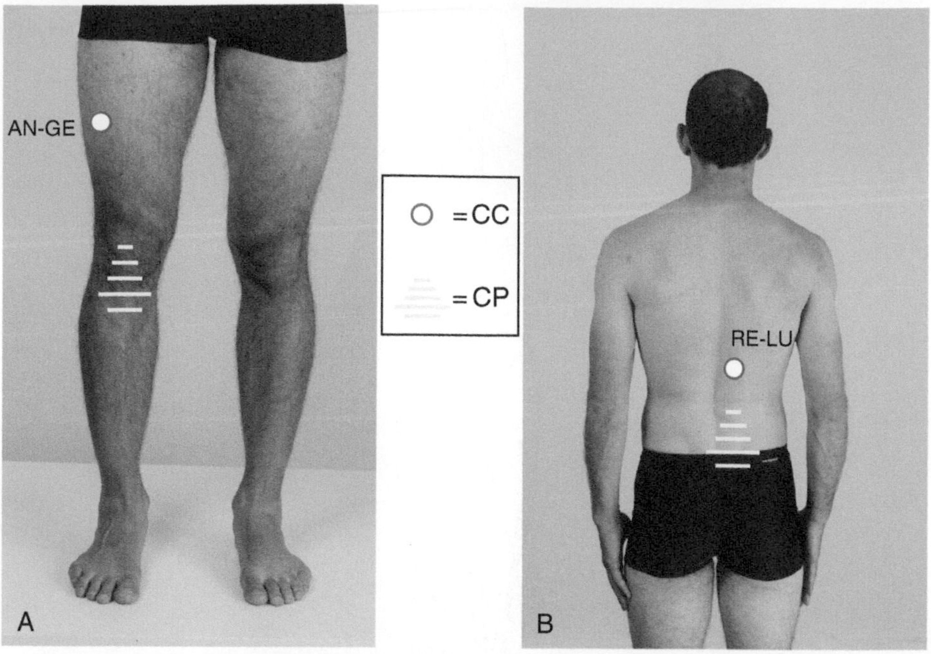

Fig. 4.10 Two examples of centres of perception. RE-LU causing pain above the sacral area and AN-GE causing pain to the anterior part of the knee, below the kneecap.

only one direction (plane). MFSs on the same spatial plane (sagittal, frontal, or horizontal) are reciprocally antagonistic. The agonist and antagonist must always be balanced or the whole spatial plane related to that MF sequence will be compromised. Due to the extensive proprioceptive fascial innervation, the sequences also have a role in monitoring upright posture in the three spatial planes.

The FM method is based on an idea of MFUs and fascial meeting points (CCs, CFs). Luigi Stecco created movement and palpation verification to highlight the problems in the myofascial system. CCs are forming lines and these lines are named after the movement direction they govern. Using this system guides the therapist towards the solution of the problem. The first step is to learn the FM language to understand method. The use of abbreviations makes the process faster and easier.

SEQUENCE OF ANTEMOTION–ANTEPULSION

Antemotion means that our body parts are moving forward in the sagittal plane. The upper extremity sequence is formed by the anatomical position, palms facing forward. The CC of AN-CU refers to elbow flexion and AN-HU shoulder flexion. CCs are found often at the intersection of muscles and fascial layers like AN-CU, which is located on the midlateral side of the biceps at the level of the deltoid muscle insertion.

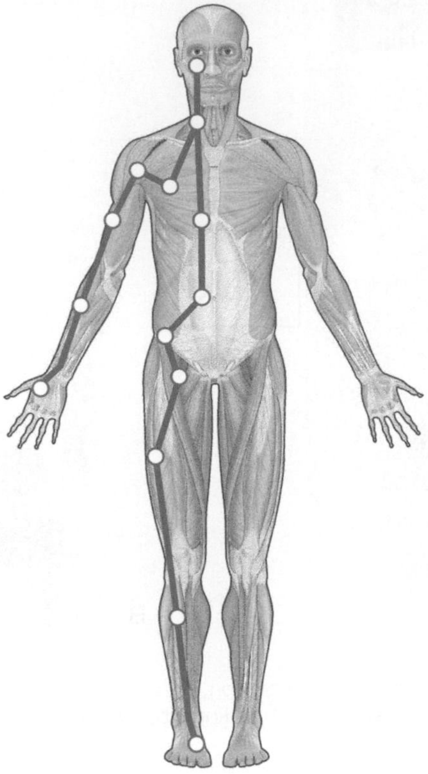

Fig. 4.11 Antemotion/antepulsion sequence.

The following is an example of common complaints relating to the anterior knee that may be associated with the antemotion fascial sequence (Fig. 4.11). Densification of AN-GE along with other CCs might be responsible for pain in the anterior part of the knee, walking downhill, or descending stairs and squatting. The CP for this point is often felt towards the knee joint. The CC, AN-GE, is formed over the rectus intermedius, located halfway down the thigh between the rectus femoris and vastus lateralis muscles. If involved, palpation of AN-GE would feel densified with a lack of fascial gliding. It would usually palpate as very tender even though the pain is around the anterior knee joint. The patient is usually completely unaware of the painful AN-GE. In the history of this GE-AN pain, the patient might have also complained of chronic pain in the iliac fascia, hip, or groin. It could be possible that the hip and groin pain preceded the knee pain. In this anterior sequence an AN-PV point might also be palpated which is located medially and slightly below the ASIS on the fascia over the iliacus muscle. Anatomically and functionally, AN-PV is important because the inguinal ligament area is the attachment point for both the abdominal muscles and thigh muscles. Maybe this patient had a previous appendectomy that affected fascia in the hip and knee. Could the knee pain be a compensatory problem due to a previous hip or even abdominal surgical trauma?

Following up the anterior sequence a therapist might find a densified AN-TH (thoracic), which is located above the lower border of the rib cage, seventh, eighth rib, where the rectus abdominis inserts and adheres to the pectoralis major muscle. The site of pain in this area is often felt as a sensation of pressure or a respiratory problem. This anterior sequence continues over the pectoralis minor muscle toward the upper limb. Anxiety can also relate to this area. The CP of this point is often located above this CC, near the sternum. The previously noted AN-HU point is also located in the anterior sequence. Alteration of this CC might cause pain in the anterior part of the shoulder and it is in some cases diagnosed as capsulitis. CP of this point is noticed over top of the shoulder, near the acromion. A shoulder pain could be related to proximal or distal points.

One example from the head area is AN-CP3 (CP, caput, skull), which can be palpated over the anterior digastric muscle belly, under the inferior border of the mandible. This point is often densified in patients who complain of clicking or pain when opening the mouth. Deviations when opening the mouth are common and the CP is often noticed in the temporomandibular (TMJ) area. Patients who are stressed can suffer from dental issues or bruxism and typically complain about these symptoms.

SEQUENCE OF RETROMOTION–RETROPULSION

Retromotion (RE) represents backward movement in the sagittal plane (Fig. 4.12). In the trunk it is a backward motion or extension from the caput and cervical spine to the pelvis. There is also of course backward movement in the upper and lower limbs. The points in the trunk are located over the erector spinae muscles from RE-CL to RE-PV. A common point often associated with chronic lumbar and lumbosacral pain is RE-LU located in the erector spinae at the level of T12–L1 or the area where the lumbar lordosis becomes kyphotic. Often symptoms are aggravated during concentric or eccentric work of the back. The CP of this area is felt in the lumbosacral region, where fascial imbalance is typically manifested. This retro sequence continues to the proximal sacrotuberous ligament (RE-CX) and to the hamstrings (RE-GE) located halfway between the gluteal fold and the popliteal fossa at the long head of the biceps femoris muscle. RE-GE is often responsible for pain (CP) in the popliteal fossa. Dysfunction of this area might over time result in popliteal cysts. Cramps may arise when flexing the knee. The retro sequence in the upper extremity travels from the infraspinatus fossa to the lateral part of the triceps to the extensor carpi ulnaris muscle ending at the RE-DI (digiti) point, which is located over abductor digiti minimi muscle towards the base of fifth metacarpal bone. Dysfunction of this area might limit hand shaking or cause pain with a closed fist. Active contraction of the abductor digiti minimi muscle may reproduce the symptoms.

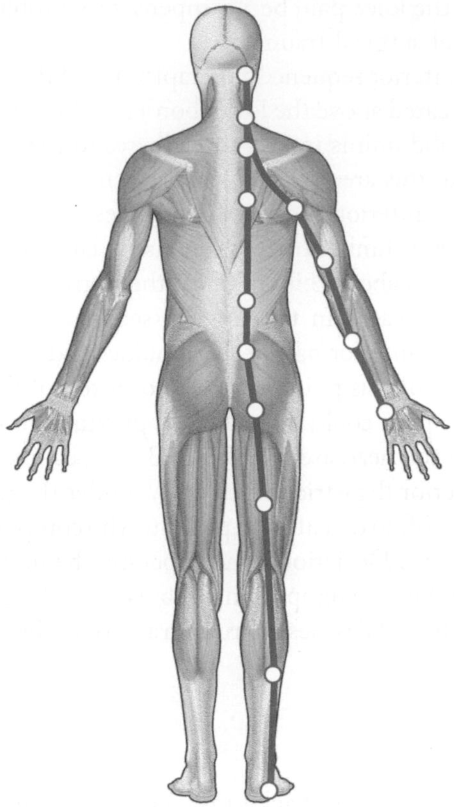

Fig. 4.12 Retromotion/retropulsion sequence.

CC of the head (caput) RE-CP3 can be involved in neck or shoulder pain. This point can be palpated in the epicranial fascia inferior and medial to the occipital protuberance. RE-CP3 may be involved with headache or dizziness. Pins and needles (paraesthesia) in the upper extremity can often be due to fascial densities along any of the upper extremity sequences.

SEQUENCE OF LATEROMOTION–LATEROPULSION

Lateromotion refers to the frontal plane: side-bending or abduction of the body (Fig. 4.13). In the lower extremity the CCs of LA-CX and LA-GE control the abduction of the hip and leg. These points are located over the tensor fascia latae muscle and halfway along the iliotibial tract near the origin of the short head of biceps femoris. In the upper extremity the CC of LA-HU is activated by abduction of the upper arm. Lateral fibres of the deltoid muscle are participating in this action. Side bending of the trunk relates to LA-LU and LA-TH CCs. The quadratus lumborum and thoracis iliocostalis muscles are affected by these points.

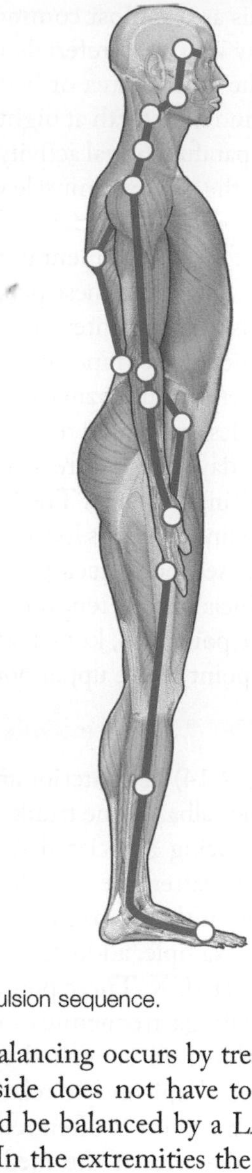

Fig. 4.13 Lateromotion/lateropulsion sequence.

In the trunk, antagonist balancing occurs by treating CCs on the opposite side, except that the opposite side does not have to be balanced at the same level. LA-LU on the right could be balanced by a LA-TH on the left if designated by palpation verification. In the extremities the balancing sequence would be a mediomotion point somewhere on the medial side of the same extremity.

LA-GE is often compromised in knee instability and the feeling of the knee giving away. The CP associated with LA-GE could be located over the fibular insertion of the iliotibial tract. Patients are typically complaining of lateral knee pain. This area is commonly overused in sports like football and running. High impacts may affect the iliotibial tract leading to imbalances, including tightness around the thigh. A common point when a patient is suffering with low back pain is LA-PV. It is located between the lateral muscle fibres of the gluteus maximus and posterior fibres of gluteus medius muscle, midway between the PSIS and greater trochanter. The CP of this area is most commonly felt along the buttock and iliotibial tract. This area may also send referrals toward the low back. The patient will report tiredness of the lumbar area or beltlike tightness.

People who are stressed and grind their teeth at night have the tendency to densify the LA-CP3 point. This oral parafunctional activity is known as bruxism. LA-CP3 can be found in the centre of the masseter muscle whose CP often refers pain towards the temporomandibular joint (TMJ). Being that the masseter muscle is one of the key motor areas of the TMJ, impairment in this area may lead to uncoordinated movements of the jaw. Quite often these people report neck or shoulder pain or even numbness in the hands. Another interesting point is LA-SC. This CC is located against the anterior border of the trapezius toward the scalenus medius. Its CP can be located along the ascending trapezius towards the neck. This point is at the junction where several muscles are located regarding the balance of the neck and shoulder girdle area. These days people are stressed by prolonged sitting behind a desk, thereby compromising this area. The lateromotion sequence ends in the upper limb at the LA-DI point, which is located over the first dorsal interosseus muscle between the first and second metacarpals. FM is used over fascia that extends between the abductor pollicis and the tendons of other fingers. In this area can also be found the acupuncture point LI4, known as *hegu* in Chinese, which is thought to be the universal pain point of the upper body.

SEQUENCE OF MEDIOMOTION–MEDIOPULSION

The mediomotion sequence (Fig. 4.14) lies anterior and posterior in the midline over the spinous processes and linea alba. In the trunk this sequence has an essentially perceptive role rather than being associated with musculoskeletal movement. In the upper and lower extremities mediomotion is an important sequence in controlling adduction of the limbs in the frontal plane and is a balancer for the lateral sequence. For example, adduction of the leg is controlled with CCs of ME-TA, ME-GE, and ME-CX. These points are located in the medial side of the lower limb over the medial gastrocnemius and adductor muscles. In the upper extremity, for example, adduction is created by ME-CU. This point is located 4 cm proximal to the medial epicondyle relating to intermuscular force transmission in the upper arm. This point is often related to tennis elbow problems. Its CP can be noticed in the area of the medial epicondyle. The upper extremity ME sequence ends medially at the hypothenar eminence.

A typically altered CC when having knee or hip problems is the ME-GE point. It is located posterior to sartorius and anterior to the gracilis muscles. You can palpate this CC four to five fingers proximal to the medial knee joint in the middle part of the thigh. CP from this area will refer to the medial area of the knee. Since the adductor muscles are controllers and stabilizers for the lower limbs, densifications at these medial points may occur after injuries or trauma. In the trunk this sequence is more perceptional, and it is often treated with CFs relating to internal dysfunction problems. Centre of coordinations of posterior mediomotion are travelling

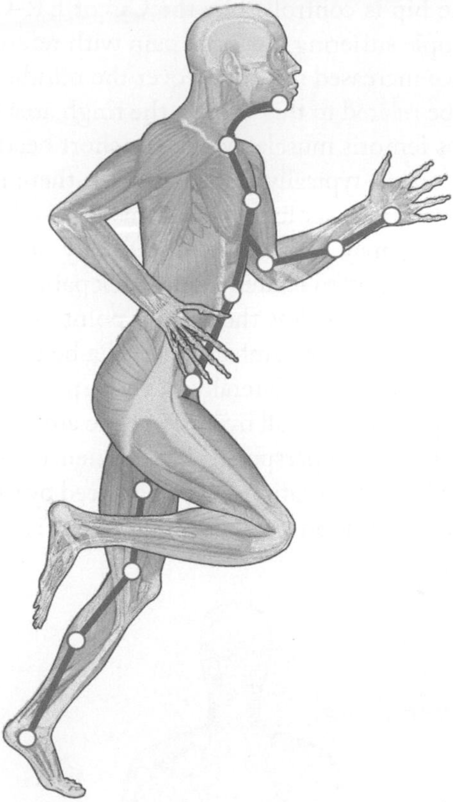

Fig. 4.14 Mediomotion/mediopulsion sequence. Mediomotion is also travelling from the occipital notch to the base of the sacral bone, in the line of processus spinosus. In the image only the anterior part of the mediomotion sequence is visualized together with the centre of coordinations of the limbs.

from occipital notch to base of the sacral bone, in the line of processus spinosus. Anterior mediomotion sequence is formed from tip of the mandibula towards the pubic bone. In the trunk area the ME-SC point relates to upper limb or shoulder girdle problems. Location of this point is at the fourth intercostal space over the clavi-coraco-axillary fascia beneath the pectoralis major tendon. Alteration of this point can relate to shoulder external pain and shoulder weakness.

Every CC sequence and CF diagonal has points located near the eye and quite often areas of the eye require treatment. Headache, vision, and hearing disturbances are indicators to palpate these points. Eye disturbances, including strabismus, might relate to ME-CP1. CP of this area is palpated at the inner corner of the eye.

SEQUENCE OF EXTRAROTATION

This sequence governs the external rotation, outer, lateral component in the horizontal plane. Rotations are typically included in most of the tasks we perform.

Lateral rotation of the hip is controlled by the CC of ER-CX, located over the piriformis muscle. People suffering low back pain with referred pain towards the lower limb often notice increased sensitivity over the middle of the buttock. Sciatic type of pain may be related to this CC. In the thigh area the ER-GE point is located over the biceps femoris muscle, where the short head originates from the lateral septum. This point is typically densified when there is referred pain from the back or lateral side of the lower limb. CP of this area is the lateral knee region. Problems with squatting may be associated. Distally along this sequence we encounter ER-PV, which is often related to low back pain. It can be palpated over the gluteus medius muscle, just below the highest point of the iliac crest. Patients usually report pain in the sacral or lumbar area and a beltlike pain, which is very typical. CP of this point is located laterally in the hip area. When treating this point a patient may report referrals all over the pelvic area from the inguinal area to the sacrum. From a treatment perspective this sequence can be balanced several ways in the trunk. Left PV extrarotation can be balanced by right PV extrarotation or left intrarotation depending on palpation findings (Fig. 4.15).

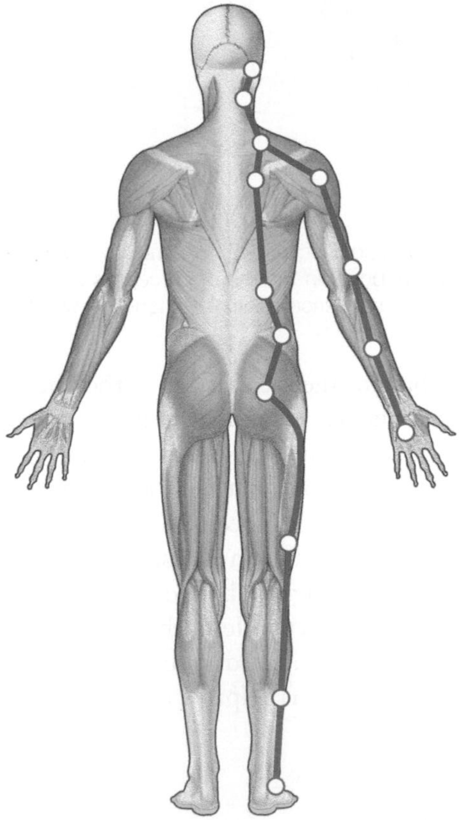

Fig. 4.15 Extrarotation sequence.

Rotation of the neck can be related to ER-CL. It is located in the level of C2/C3 where the levator scapulae muscle inserts. Problems in the neck and lumbar area involving rotational components are often involved. Patients complain of pain upon turning the head or trying to rotate the neck backwards. Closely related to neck and shoulder girdle pain is ER-SC. It is located in the belly of the levator scapulae muscle, above the superior angle of the scapula. This point has a CP around the neck area. Testing for asynchrony between the scapula and humerus may be positive. Patients note symptoms of this CC as pain in the neck or shoulder. Referred paraesthesia toward the hands is possible.

Continuing toward the upper limb we encounter the ER-HU point. It is located over the distal part of infraspinatus and teres minor muscles and posterior fibres of the deltoid muscle. This area is an important intersection when working with the upper limbs: lifting, holding, pushing, or pulling. CP of this point is often described as pain around the glenohumeral joint. Examination of the upper extremity may show that supination of the forearm is associated with the ER-CA CC. This point is over the extensor digitorum and extensor pollicis longus muscles. Injuries of the wrist and forearm might lead to involvement of the shoulder area. Prolonged problems may cause cysts over the extensor tendons. This horizontal sequence ends at the dorsal fascia of the hand at the third and fourth or fourth and fifth metacarpals: ER-DI.

From the head area we can highlight meaningful points associated with upper neck problems, including vertigo, tinnitus, and headaches. The point ER-CP3 is located over the mastoid notch and is in continuity with the posterior auricular muscle. CP of this area is often felt in the forehead.

SEQUENCE OF INTRAROTATION

The intrarotation sequence contains inward, medial or internal rotation movement of the horizontal plane (Fig. 4.16). This sequence works as a balance for the extrarotation sequence. One example of intrarotation in the lower limb is inward rotation of the hip. This motion is governed by CC of IR-CX, located at the angle of the femoral triangle. Another example of the lower limb focuses on the IR-GE point. It is located over the muscle belly of vastus medialis obliquus and typically relates to knee pain. CP of this point is the medial region of the knee and is associated with medial meniscus and medial collateral ligament lesions.

In the trunk, the intrarotation sequence travels from IR points of PV, LU, and TH up to the two heads of sternocleidomastoideus. In that area is the IR-CL point, which participates in internal rotation of the neck. This area relates to torticollis and difficulty in turning the head. Neck, thorax, and lumbar movements are balanced by extrarotation points. Rotation of the thorax to the left can be balanced by intratotation on the left side with extrarotation on the right side. In the lumbar area IR-LU point is at the tip of 11th rib over the external oblique muscle. Rotation of the lumbar or thoracic spine might be reduced with complaints of

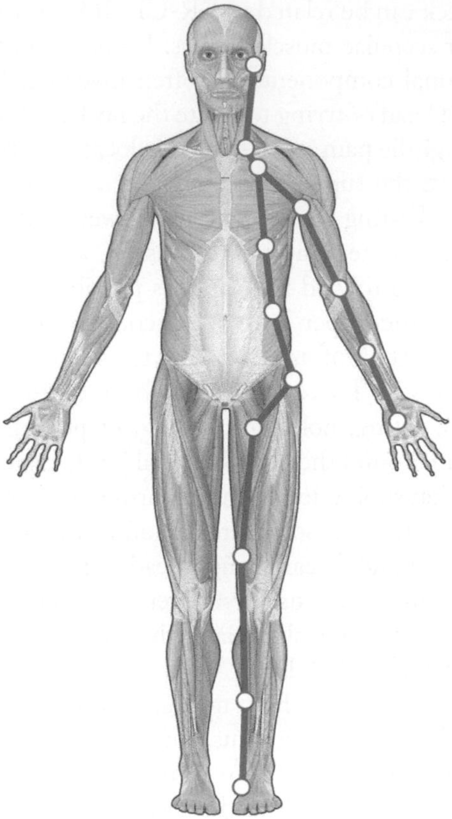

Fig. 4.16 Intrarotation sequence.

pain in the abdominal or inguinal regions. Breathing problems and pain in the ribcage might also arise from the IR-TH area. The CC is palpated in the fifth or sixth intercostal spaces below the nipple. Skipping to the head is IR-CP3 where densification may be responsible for bruxism, stress, and eating problems. This point is located in the sulcus behind the mandible, between the earlobe and the neck of the mandible. The CP of this point is around the TMJ. Moving from the head toward the upper limb travelling over to the subclavius muscle we can identify the IR-SC point beneath the middle third of the clavicle. This point often refers pain to the medial head of the clavicle.

The intrarotation sequence toward the upper limb begins from the IR-HU point, located beneath pectoralis major and coracoclavicular fascia. The intersection of many muscles can create fascial tension in this area creating pain anterior to the glenohumeral joint. The CC of IR-CU might become altered with overuse of the forearm from homework or repairing things. It is located over the pronator teres, which participates in rotational movements. The medial epicondyle is a typical place to where pain often refers. This IR sequence ends at the palm of the hand on the palmaris longus at the intercarpal space below the second to fourth metacarpals. In the palm area fascia is not free to slide, as it is more involved in grasping and holding so densification in this area is usually associated with using tools and injuries of the fingers or wrist. CC sequences need help from CFs, diagonals, and spirals to maintain function in everyday life and in tasks requiring fine motor tuning and proprioception. For this combination we now turn to the CFs.

Centres of Fusion (see Video 11)

Flexing of the shoulder joint represents movement in the sagittal plane. The force is created and controlled by specific MFUs capable of activating that movement beginning with the MFU AN-HU, which is located in the anterior part of the deltoid muscle, medial to the long heads of the biceps tendon. When the upper extremity flexes as a unit with simultaneous movement of the elbow and wrist joints, a whole line of MFUs are activated. The adjoining CCs along this line are called a sequence. But movements, as we know, do not occur only along single planes. We only move our arm, for example, in an anterior or lateral direction. Luigi Stecco realized this and discovered what are called CFs. The CFs represent the intermediate ranges of movement between the unilateral sequences. CFs are at the site where two single-plane MFUs converge in order to synchronize the action of two related MFUs. They are located in the aponeurotic fascia in the crossing of different fascial planes. They guarantee gradualism, harmony, and modulation during the passage between two movement directions.

While CCs act more with muscle spindles, CFs relate more with Golgi tendon organs and Ruffini and Pacini corpuscles. For example, AN-LA-HU (CF of anterior-lateral-humerus) controls all the intermediate movements between the MFU of anterior shoulder movement and the MFU of lateral shoulder movement. Actually, almost all of our functions, daily tasks, and movements are not happening in unilateral anatomical planes but rather somewhere in between. That is why we need the cooperation of all anatomical planes and the ability to generate force and control movement between sequences. An important reason for the CF is that in the intermediate movement, in this example, it is very possible that the LA-HU MFU may be more active than the AN-HU MFU. In other words, there might be increased activity in one MFU and decreased activity in an associated MFU. This represents an uncoordinated situation or what some call an accident waiting to happen. For no apparent reason a tennis player complains of shoulder pain in external rotation, which can be caused by uncoordinated receptors stuck in the fascia. Of course the densification of AN-LA-HU could be happening because of a previous trauma to the elbow or wrist with densifications in the wrist (AN-LA-CA) or elbow (AN-LA-CU). Therefore an important function of the CF is to coordinate or balance the intermediate muscle fibres that are activated during movement between the MFUs of two planes. The shoulder joint is a ball-and-socket joint able to move through 360° including all anatomical planes and all planes between them. Because CFs are related to complex movements, a rotational element is always inferred, so treatment of the horizontal plane is always included if necessary with treatment of CF planes.

The AN-ME sequence is another example where there may be more or less activity in either the anterior or medial MFU sequence (Fig. 4.17). Because functional movements always include rotational components, a third needed vector is included. Between AN and ME there is a, MFU called IR-HU (intrarotation humerus), which is located beneath the pectoralis major, on the coracoclavicular and subscapularis fascia. According to movement analysis AN relates to flexion and ME to adduction. IR-HU produces movement in medial rotation. Combining

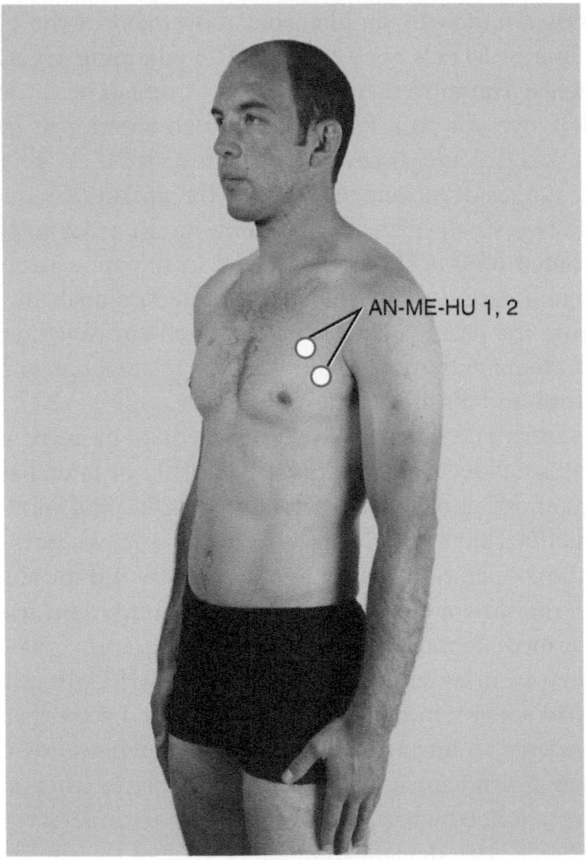

Fig. 4.17 Centre of fusion of AN-ME-HU located over the thoracic border of the axillary retinaculum. From here it organizes the synergy between pectoralis major, coracobrachialis, and latissimus dorsi.

these three MFUs creates an AN-ME direction. Thinking of the joint and its articular functions, when the arm is moving toward flexion (AN) and adduction (ME), there has to be an associated medial rotation (IR), otherwise this movement would not be possible. CFs are created in the junction of two sequences (Box 4.4). This kind of joint movement and simultaneous gliding–rolling action has been described by several authors in the history of manipulative treatments (Banks and Hengeveld, 2013; Cyriax, 1984; Kaltenborn and Evjenth, 2002; Maitland et al., 2001).

The Diagonal System of Movement

CFs are formed along lines similar to CCs. CC lines are called sequences and CF lines are called diagonals. There are four diagonal lines: two anterior, AN-ME and AN-LA, and two posterior, RE-ME and RE-LA. These diagonals are derived from two adjacent CC sequences. Diagonals unite unidirectional CFs. The diagonal line corresponds to movement occurring between sequences (Fig. 4.19). This organization is similar to Herman Kabat's ideas of proprioceptive neuromuscular facilitation (PNF) movements, which also work along four diagonal directions. PNF rehabilitation focuses on diagonal pattern activation rather than single-muscle activation (Adler et al., 2008). Activation of diagonal patterns is a way of demonstrating how the human brain works regarding movement. Stecco (2004) discussed these ideas based on the directional basis of movement rather than on an individual muscle basis. Stecco wrote that the force of contraction is based primarily on the number of motor units stimulated and that the CNS does not recognize single muscle activity. The CNS recognizes only general movements.

The CFs along diagonals form a fusion line between CC sequences. CFs fine-tune motor control and influence the amount of force generation of MFUs. Most of our daily tasks, like picking up a glass of water, require many MFUs in many

BOX 4.4

CCs are located mostly over the muscle bellies and they interact with muscle spindles. They synchronize forceful unidirectional movements. They are recruited when effort or force is required and when the muscle attachments to the fascia are under tension.

CFs are located over retinacula and periarticular structures, near joints, over tendons, and in the trunk along lines of union of some muscles. See the retinaculum area in wrist (Fig. 4.18). CFs interact with Golgi tendon organs that provide feedback dealing with muscle force, joint position, and direction. They are recruited by stretching of retinacula either directly (via tendons) or indirectly (via movements of bones onto which they are inserted). The CF therefore is the site where two different myofascial units (MFUs) converge in order to synchronize the action of two MFUs. It is located in the aponeurotic fascia in the crossing of different fascial planes. It guarantees gradualism, harmony, and modulation during the passage between two movement directions (Stecco, 2004).

Continued

BOX 4.4 —cont'd

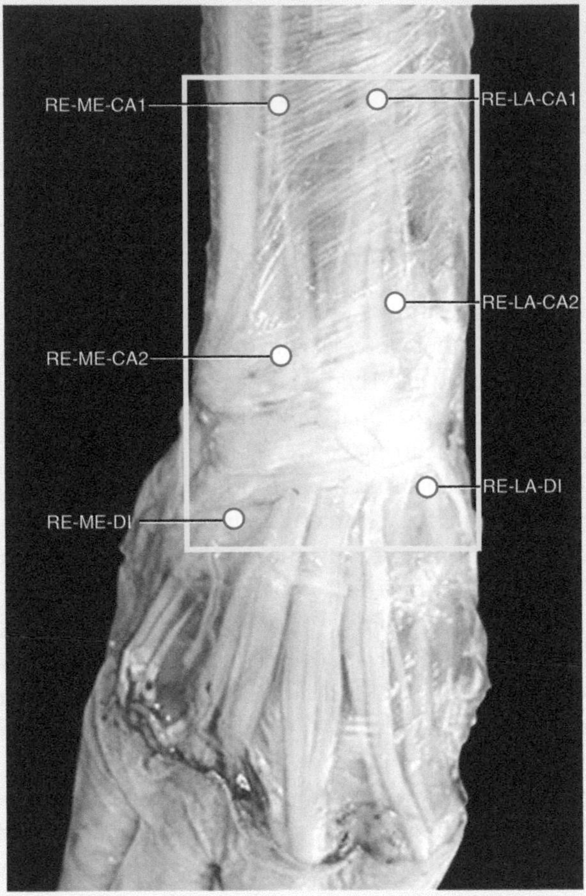

Fig. 4.18 Centre of fusions of dorsal side of the wrist. *(From Stecco, 2015.)*

different planes associated with nearby segments. Therefore, the need for a diagonal line of force is obvious. If we use only MFUs for daily tasks, we would first raise an upper arm within one anatomical plane, then transfer it laterally to another plane. The movements would be angular or even square-like rather than functional. Robots have these angular like movements because coded algorithms have been programmed into their hard drives. Humans require fine-tuning and coactivation of the whole myofascial system.

When reaching with an arm, we use only that amount of force that is needed and the force is never generated only by a single MFU sequence. According to angles and lines of movement we use appropriate MFUs and only a particular

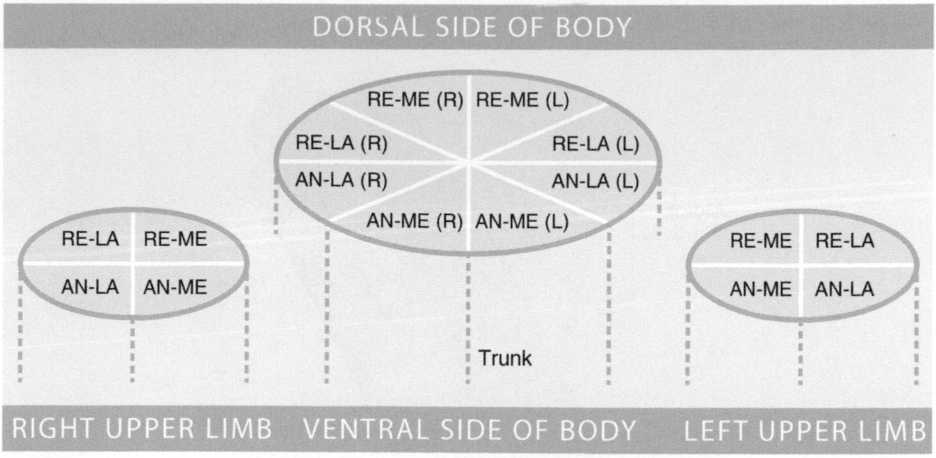

Fig. 4.19 Cake of centre of fusions diagonals.

amount of them are necessary for proper movement (see Box 4.5). Via CFs our CNS is able to fade forces of the MFUs in and out in appropriate degrees, resulting in smooth and coordinated movement. This is an example where our brain coordinates movement with the help of CCs and uses CFs for fine-tuning.

When we move forward by walking, movement seems to occur in the sagittal plane. But walking itself is a complex mix of different functions including many segments and different planes. While moving forward along a sagittal plane, in every step weight transfers along the frontal plane from one side to other and simultaneously the horizontal plane is activated allowing rotational movement. In the lower and upper limbs CFs are arranged in four diagonals: AN-ME, AN-LA, RE-ME, and RE-LA. Walking and gait can be described kinematically as heel strike, midphase, and toe off. A foot lands on the ground (heel strike) and continues to the midphase, where the body shifts weight over the foot and the whole leg, while other leg swings forward to start a new contact phase. During weight transfer the body is moving forward and laterally. Hip joint movement occurs at the same time in retromotions and mediomotions. Especially in

BOX 4.5

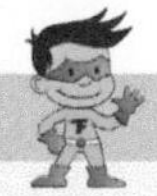

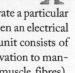

Motor units are activated with the "all-or-none rule." The motor neurons innervate a particular amount of muscle cells (fibres), typically about 100 to 200 for most muscles. When an electrical stimulus arrives via the nerve, all of its muscle cells are activated. A myofascial unit consists of many motor units that activate separately. Actually, people use only enough activation to manage a motor task. A gamma nerve regulates muscle spindle cells (intrafusal muscle fibres), which eventually regulate extrafusal muscle contraction as needed. This action is more reflex based and can happen without direct motor cortex involvement (Fig. 4.20).

Continued

BOX 4.5 ■ **—cont'd**

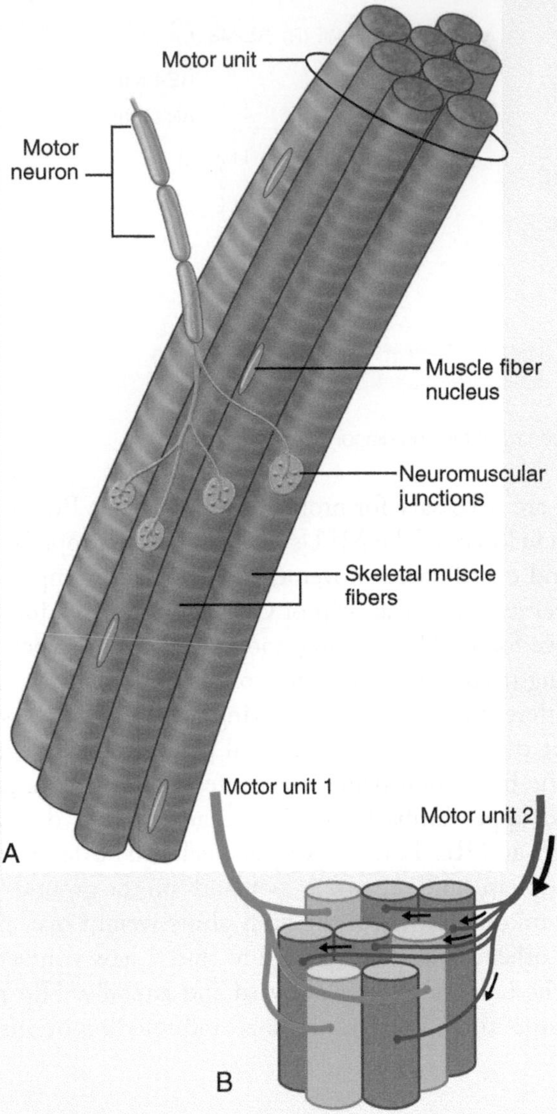

Fig. 4.20 Activation of motor unit.

segments COXA and GENU (hip and knee joint) the diagonal RE-ME takes control. Immediately after the first contact, the RE sequence is more responsible to generate force, but the action of the ME motion (adduction of hip) is dependent on the amount of frontal plane movement. As previously discussed in the example of the hand and reaching, and also in gait, the movement should be

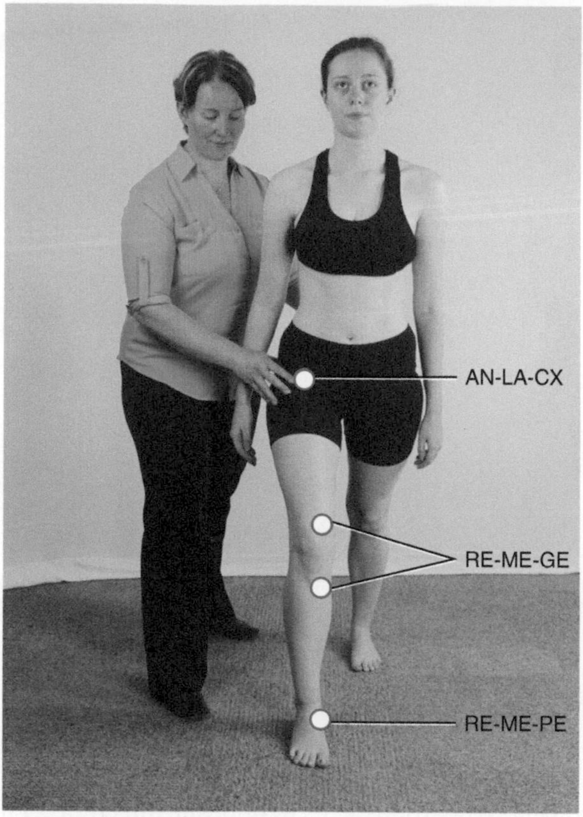

Fig. 4.21 Assessment of stepping forward.

smooth. The CFs RE-ME-GE and RE-ME-CX are fine-tuning forces between RE and ME motions.

For example, if a patient complains of pain when walking, the densified points might be located in RE-ME diagonal in the lower extremity and the anterior and lateral part of the upper thigh, AN-LA-CX could work as a balancing point for the FM treatment in this case (Fig. 4.21). This is just one part of gait cycle; the rest of the gait cycle is discussed later with spiral function.

The Spiral System of Movement: Control and Fine-Tuning for Optimal Performance

Spirals represent the sum of the helicoidal tensions that the CFs create in the fascia. They are necessary for the regulation of complex motor activities or movements like walking (Stecco, 2004). Spirals unite CFs in particular formations to account for complex movements such as swimming or running and most athletic movements involving bilateral use of the body. They are responsible, along with CC sequences, for the accumulation of energy dealing with the facilitation of

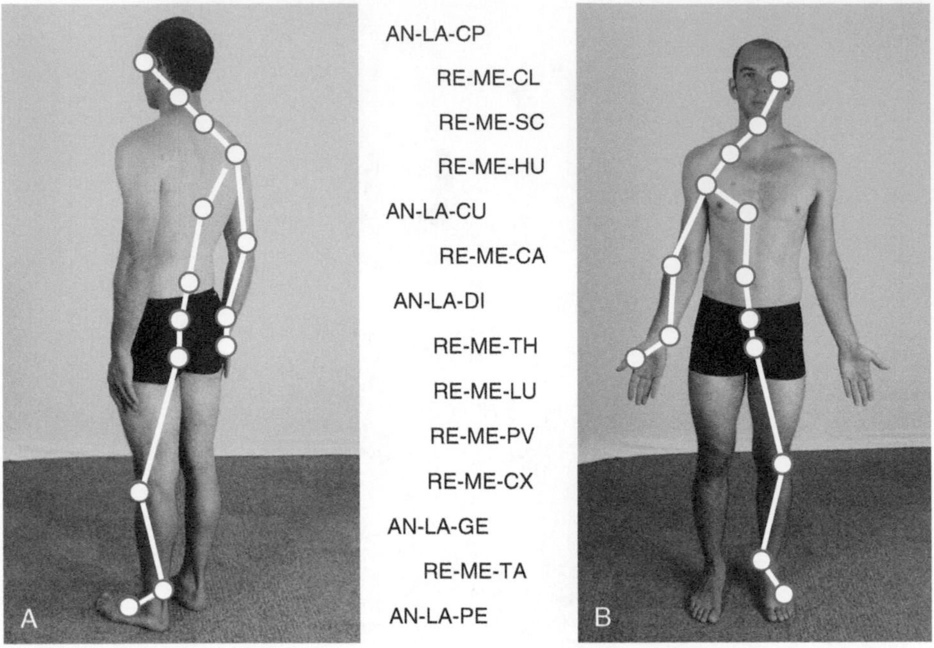

Fig. 4.22 Example of spiral, AN-LA.

force and countermovement as energy is released during dynamic movement. Spirals, as explained later, synchronize CFs in opposite directions. They are involved in the coordination of complex motor patterns, or opposite actions between two or more adjacent segments (Fig. 4.22).

In the lower extremities there are four spiral pathways of CFs. They are named, for example, using the CFs of the PES segment (foot) (Stecco, 2004): RE-LA-PE, RE-ME-PE, AN-LA-PE, and AN-ME-PE (Fig. 4.23). Spirals usually originate from termination areas such as the foot, head, or hand travelling via the torso (also can originate from next proximal area such as the talus or carpi). Four diagonals AN-LA, AN-ME and RE-LA, RE-ME are also present in the upper extremities just as described for the lower limbs.

Spirals in the trunk arise from the head. The head acts as a motor guide for the whole trunk. The CFs form two diagonals on both sides of the body. In the anterior part there exists AN-LA and AN-ME diagonals on both sides of the linea alba. Posteriorly the RE-LA and RE-ME diagonals are also on both sides of the spinous processes. Spirals are also described in the trunk, where they connect diagonals of CFs to functional movement patterns (Fig. 4.24).

Spirals allow us to control and produce force in complex movements while walking or performing a skilful act. For instance, martial arts kicking demands at the same time both high velocity force generation and good flexibility. In the gait cycle different segments move in opposite ways. While the ankle is

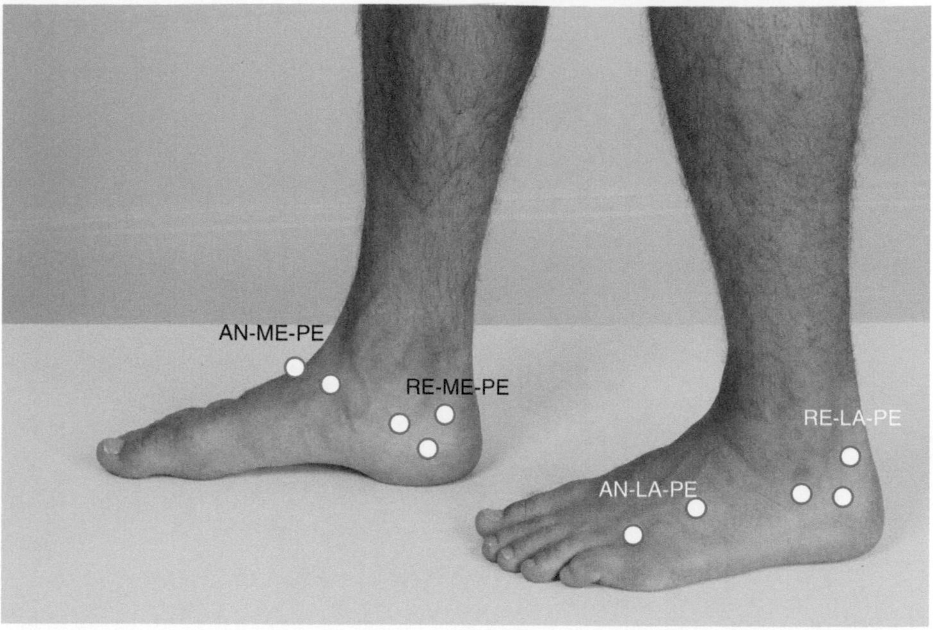

Fig. 4.23 Starting points of the spirals. The spiral of the RE-LA-PE arises from the posterior and lateral portion of calcaneal area heading toward the medial and anterior portion of shin area. The spiral of RE-ME-PE arises also from the posterior side of the calcaneal area but medially relative to the RE-LA-PE spiral's origin. From the medial side it travels over to the lateral and anterior side of the shin. The spiral of the AN-LA-PE arises at the anterior and lateral portion of the foot travelling toward the medial posterior side of the shin, near the Achilles tendon. The fourth spiral is the AN-ME-PE arising from the anterior and medial side of the foot near the area of insertion of the tibialis anterior muscle. From there it goes to the posterior side of the shin, lateral side of the Achilles tendon.

moving towards dorsiflexion (antemotion) the knee joint is moving toward flexion (retromotion) while the hip joint moves toward flexion (antemotion). Attempting to independently control all those segments and their movements in opposing ways would be a mission impossible or, at the very least, that kind of movement would be very slow or angular-like. Therefore, a spiral-like-system is the only reasonable solution; it can control in one "line" both agonist and antagonist motion along the whole musculoskeletal system.

Examples of Spiral Movements

WALKING

Gait is a basic human motion. Since the days of Aristotle, humans have been trying to understand and observe walking, stepping, and gait. Still, in present days there are a lot of arguments on how to observe gait or how to analyse and define heel strike or midfoot strike. For optimal gait it is important to understand that the

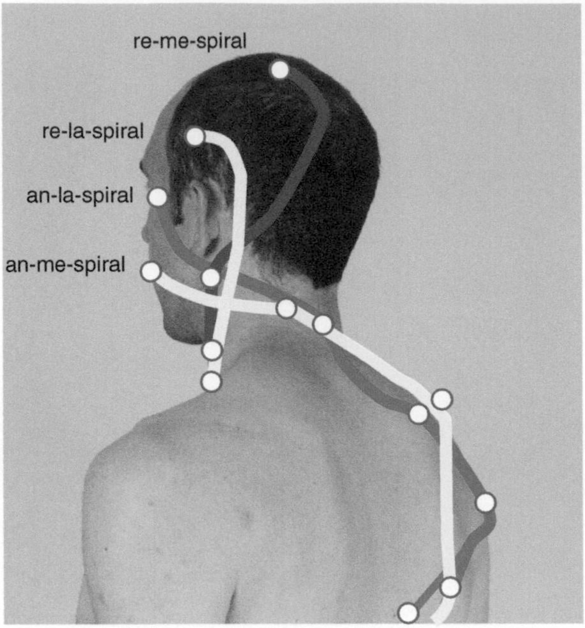

Fig. 4.24 Spirals in the head.

whole body is moving while walking, not only the feet. The feet and ankle move, but also the knee, hip, pelvis, spine, rib cage, and upper arms. All segments are necessary and a disorder in any segment may cause consequences and misalignments in other segments affecting gait. A disorder in one segment can affect an entire movement pattern, such as reduced knee flexion range in patients with a reconstructed anterior cruciate ligament (Shi et al., 2010). Errors in gait patterns (sometimes called pathological gait patterns) most often result from musculoskeletal problems including stiffness, pain, or joint misalignment. There may also be neurological conditions (multiple sclerosis, cerebral palsy, amyotrophic lateral sclerosis, etc.), congenital abnormalities, or other diseases that affect our movements (Fig. 4.25).

Some authors define walking as a controlled falling forward and others state that locomotion is the translation of the centre of gravity along a pathway

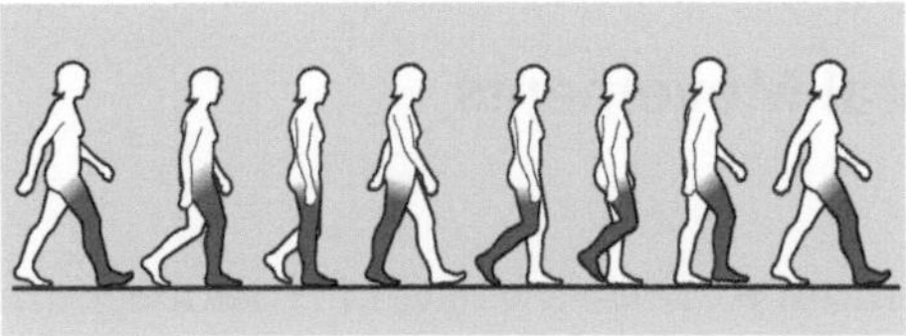

Fig. 4.25 Walking cycle.

requiring the least expenditure of energy (Vaughan, 2003). *Physiopedia* (2015) lists the sequences for walking as follows:

- Registration and activation of the gait command within the CNS
- Transmission of the gait system to the peripheral nervous system
- Contraction of muscles
- Generation of several forces
- Regulation of joint forces and moments across synovial joints and skeletal segments
- Generation of ground reaction forces

It becomes clear that the generation of forces (especially in functional movement) requires many segments and anatomical planes. MFUs are not capable of handling all the force generation necessary in walking. It was previously stated that the CFs help to create a smooth fusion of these forces. The CFs (diagonals), however, are not the full answer for the absorption of these forces. As stated, MFU sequences create forces along anatomical planes, and diagonals represent intermediate planes between the MFUs. Together there are overall 10 lines (six MFUs and four CFs). In walking, CC sequences and CF diagonals cannot account for all the variations that occur, for example, in the gait cycle. In the gait cycle during midstance, the ankle is in dorsiflexion (antemotion), the knee is in flexion (retromotion), and the hip is in flexion (antemotion), while at the same time a lateral force occurs due to weight transfer (lateromotion or mediomotion). With natural pelvic rotation via the horizontal plane, rotational forces are present in the entire lower leg (intra- or extramotion).

KICKING

Taekwondo is a Korean martial art and Olympic sport that includes variations of kicking, blocking, and punching techniques. All of these techniques should be performed with high velocity and accuracy. Velocity requires speed and accuracy since timing and aiming power is essential for positive acts in any combat sport. In Taekwondo and other martial arts, aiming, velocity, and power techniques are practiced, demonstrated, and tested by a special breaking technique referred to in the Korean language as *kyukpa*. Practicing begins with a soft target and proceeds to small, thin boards and then to thicker, larger, and stronger wooden and stone target-like bricks. A side-kick (in Korean, *yop chagi*) is very typical in Taekwondo; it demonstrates power and will (Fig. 4.26). At the same time, it is a brilliant example of a three-dimensional helicoidal force generation. The kick starts with raising the kicking leg's knee up in front and simultaneously turning the standing leg laterally to open the pelvic area and hip joint. This allows more free space to move with maximum flexibility at the end of the range of hip and pelvic motion. Raising a knee is actually a movement of hip flexion (antemotion), but because at the same time the supporting or standing leg is rotating from the hip

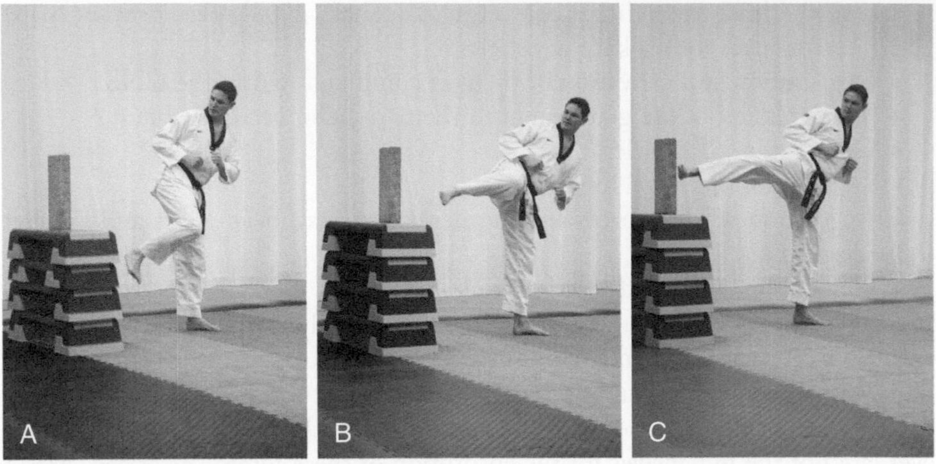

Fig. 4.26 Crushing a brick by using sidekick.

and pelvis laterally (extrarotation), the movement is not a pure antemotion but rather a motion toward flexion and abduction. Also if a joint is moving via two axes there has to be rotation, in this case, lateral rotation. This movement is AN-LA-motion of coxa (hip). The kick continues by extending a kicking leg toward the target and at the same time dorsiflexion of the ankle is preparing the impact. In other words, the hip will be abducted more (lateromotion) and simultaneously it is extended (retromotion), the knee is extended fully (antemotion), and the ankle is dorsiflexing (antemotion).

Pure power of the kick is initiated primarily by hip extension and secondarily by knee and ankle extension. The ankle movement is contradictory compared to walking. The most interesting thing about kicking and the helicoidal fascial system is the knowledge derived on how to perform a very powerful kick. One of the main principles in creating maximum power in Taekwondo is to use rotational effort. In a side kick, it is advised to use strong medial rotation while extending the knee and hip joints. This rotation should be like a bullet in a rifle, which takes maximal rotation from the rifle grooves and with rotational movement increases speed and accuracy. Experience and practice over the past thousands of years have led Korean Taekwondo masters to study movement. They understood that human movement is not just an anatomical apparatus with three planes (sagittal, frontal, and horizontal), but also functional and existing in all planes (CCs, CFs, and spirals).

LIFTING

An interesting example of the spiral system is lifting something from the ground. When we lift a bag or a similar object we grab it with the fingers and while lifting it up we extend our glenohumeral joint (shoulder joint) and

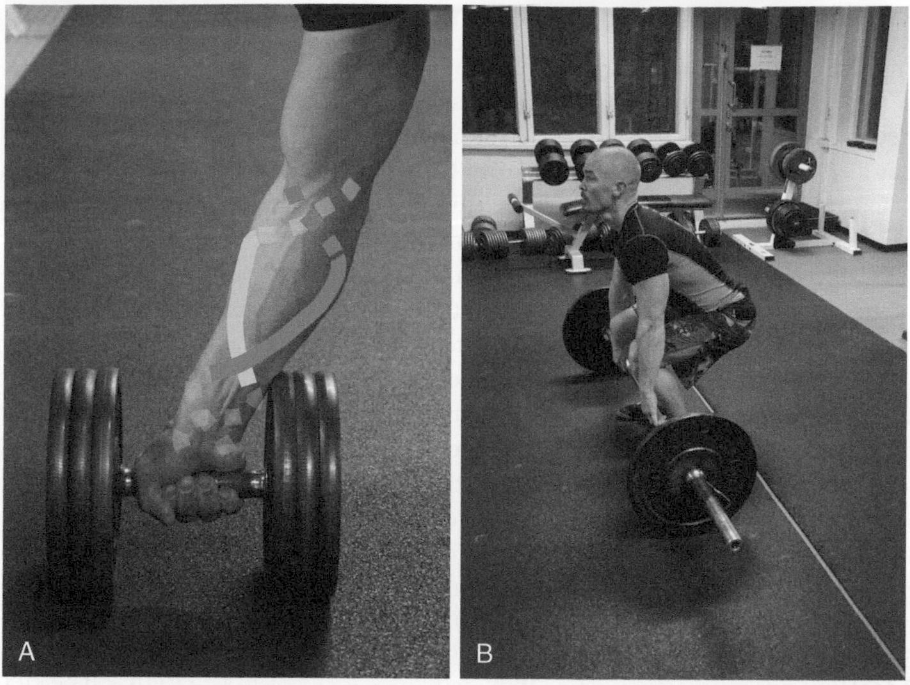

Fig. 4.27 Lifting with spiral.

flex the elbow joint. A principle in lifting is that the lever needs support strong enough to be able to lift something. This law of physics applies to human motion. The support for shoulder and upper limb is created from the trunk and if we stand while lifting, the tension from the lower limbs becomes crucial to hold the pelvis and torso stable, allowing the shoulder and upper limb to perform its action (Fig. 4.27).

The activated spiral depends on the position of the weight to be lifted. Is it on the ground or do you have to reach across to grab it? If lifting the weight from the ground near our feet, we will first engage our AN-ME-DI spiral and continue the movement activating the RE-LA-CA from the posterior and lateral side of the elbow. Activation continues toward the AN-ME-CU following the spiral to the posterior and lateral side of the shoulder, RE-LA-HU, to RE-LA-SC and RE-LA-TH. At this point the spiral is changing sides toward the contralateral RE-LA-LU and RE-LA-PV. It is evident that our movement requires a combination of different sequences, diagonal, and spirals and that we are using our bodies in individual ways. For this reason the problems people encounter vary and the therapist should be skilful when assessing and palpating the patient.

Fascial Manipulation: Treatment Protocol

The main idea of the FM protocol is to highlight that every patient is unique. Just because two patients have similar symptoms does not at all indicate that they require a similar treatment. FM is a method based on particular guidelines that lead to individualized findings and treatment procedures. The patient is in focus from the very beginning. The initial visit consists of a patient history-taking, use of an assessment chart, and an examination. From the history the therapist forms a hypothesis, which will lead to the particular related segments that require examination. Questions about the history of the present pain may include: Is this the first time that this pain ever appeared? How long has the patient had the pain? Does the pain appear on weight-bearing or at rest? There are many other questions that are necessary to ask. Past injuries or operations may relate to a current complaint. A very important question is, is there some sort of recent traumatic reason for the local pain or did the pain appear for no apparent reason? The therapist must determine if the painful site is compensating for a previous problem elsewhere or is a local issue. History-taking in FM always emphasizes the fascial kinetic chain. After forming a hypothesis, movement and palpatory verifications are performed on the chosen segments relating to the patient's complaint. In movement verification (MOVE) every movement in all the planes are tested. It is helpful to ask patients what movement bothers them the most in order to check the progress of treatment. Palpatory verification (PAVE) will be the last and most important aspect of an FM examination. Palpation determines which of the ten pathways will require treatment. Is it a sequence, diagonal, spiral, or a combination of the three? If palpation disagrees with a painful movement direction, palpation determines the line of treatment.

Treatment is guided by the knowledgeable hands and the points are chosen with care according to palpatory verification findings. Treatment is performed with fingers, knuckles, or elbows until the release is felt by both therapist and patient. When treating musculoskeletal problems, approximately six to eight points are treated per session and results should occur immediately after treatment. Assessment of the progress of a patient is done during and after treatment. After treating two or three points, has there been an improvement in motion testing (MOVE)? In the first treatment the most densified and painful plane will be treated. It is not recommended to treat more than one plane per visit since, upon the second visit, if several planes were treated, how would we know which plane was responsible for a positive response? In the second treatment session depending on the results, the same plane might be treated again or if there is absolutely no change another plane might be treated. Decisions are always based on improvement in motion and palpation (Fig. 4.28).

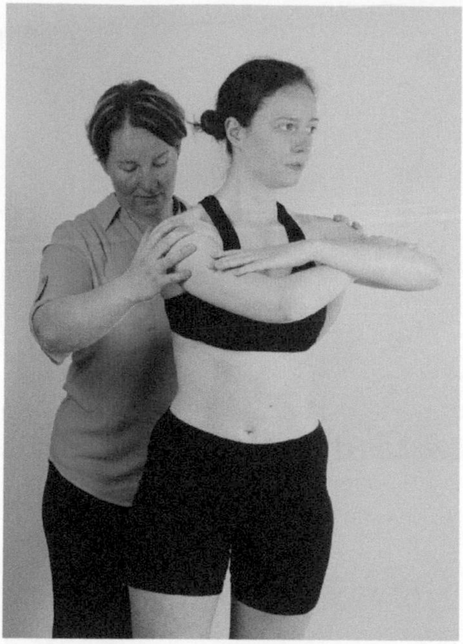

Fig. 4.28 Fascial manipulation treatment is a protocol including variable elements.

CASE HISTORY: INTERVIEW (see Video 12)

The case history is a very important part of FM. It guides the practitioner to determine the hypothesis as to what needs to be treated. The therapist has to focus on guiding the patient during the interview with regard to the main complaint and other concurrent pain and establish a time line as to what injuries, traumas, or surgeries occurred in the past. Sometimes picking up the key elements will take time. The use of the assessment chart created by FM will help with the interview process and guide the mind of the therapist to collect the pertinent data (Fig. 4.29).

The first question to ask is where is the site of pain? At times patients blurt out their whole history in a random manner. It is necessary for the therapist to control the conversation and build a timeline as to the sequence of events that might be related to the main pain. You have to find out the exact location of the pain, how and when it happened, and how much it is bothering the patient (Fig. 4.30).

All the information can be gathered on the assessment chart (Fig. 4.31). The main problem is recorded as a site of pain (SiPa). For example LU RE means lumbar area (segment) and back side (location). Side is recorded next, left, right, or bilateral. History of the problem is very important. Did the problem arise after some event, trauma, or repetitive action or stress? Or did it appear gradually? Is the problem at the moment constant or recurrent? For example, is the problem

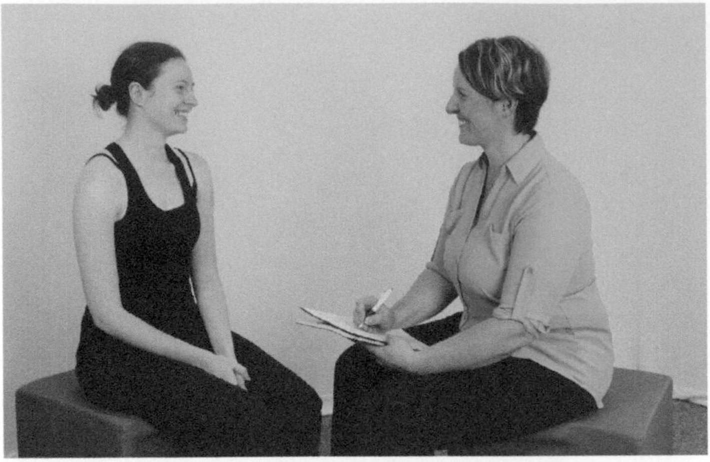

Fig. 4.29 Case history.

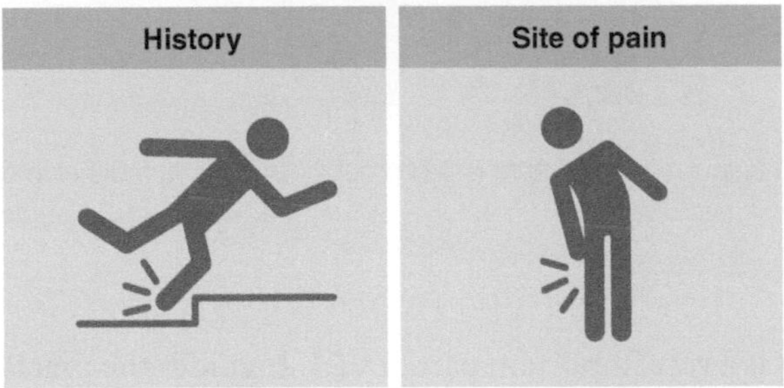

Fig. 4.30 History-taking and site of pain.

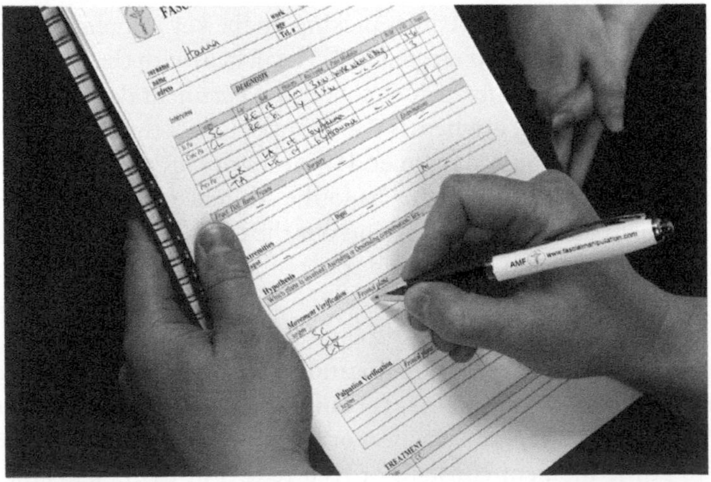

Fig. 4.31 Assessment chart.

TABLE 4.1 ■ **Assessment Chart: Site of Pain (SiPa)**

	Segment	Location	Side	History	Rec/ const	Pain Modality	Notes
SiPa	LU	RE	lt	Trauma	Const	VAS 4/10	Worse → sitting

Fascial manipulation records all the information in an economical way. From this we can determine that the patient is complaining of pain in the lumbar region, over the erector spinae muscles on the left side, caused by trauma 2 years ago and that it is constant, with a visual analogue score (VAS) of 4/10 that increases when the patient is sitting.

disturbing daily life once a week (1 × w) or three times per month, or is it always present (const)? Pain modality means things that are aggravating the symptoms, like prolonged sitting, driving, or standing. The visual analogue scale (VAS) is commonly used to measure a patient's sensation and feeling about pain on a 1 to 10 scale. Therapists might require additional pages necessary for other information, such as imaging reports and lab tests (Table 4.1).

Concomitant pain (ConcPa) is determined next. Does the patient have another complaint somewhere else, for example, in the thoracic area? Where is the exact location of this pain? The same information is needed about concomitant pain as the site of pain: segment, location, side, history, recurrences, pain modality, VAS, and additional notes. Previous pain (PrevPa) might bring to light the origin of the problem. The history might show that the patient suffered severe injuries that are not bothering him at the present time but that the recovery process persisted longer than usual. All kinds of complications or prolonged healing processes should be noted; they may be the origin of the present problem. What was the first significant pain episode and how long did it persist? Patients are masters in forgetting things. Therapists should ask direct questions to help them to remember. Have you ever been a patient in a hospital? Why? Have you ever been on sick leave for a while? Do you remember if you hurt yourself badly when you were a child? All of these direct questions might help your patients recall past happenings. Quite often at the second appointment they remark: "Hey, now I remember that I had this really bad ankle sprain when I was 15 years old. This came to my mind after the last treatment session, when my low back pain improved." People in pain may have difficulty remembering the past. With pain their mind becomes blurred and when the pain lessens, they are able to focus better about their past history (Table 4.2).

Fractures, dislocations, injuries, and operations are also recorded on the assessment chart. In addition, note examinations, imaging results, blood tests, etc., which can be meaningful when assessing the patient. Diseases and contraindications and precautions for medications should be recorded. Quite often the

TABLE 4.2 ■ Assessment Chart: Concomitant Pain (ConcPa) and Previous Pain (PrevPa)

	Segment	Location	Side	History	Rec/ const	Pain Modality	Notes
ConcPa	TH	RE	lt	?	Const	VAS 2/10	–
PrevPa	GE	AN	lt	Trauma 4 years	Not now	–	–

Recordings indicate that the thorax area from the back and left side is painful constantly. History is not known and the VAS is 2.

therapist is able to do something to relieve the pain or help the patient to move better or perform better, although there might be some underlying disease. FM treatment can often help in decreasing the amount of medication by improving homeostasis so that the body can heal itself (Table 4.3; Box 4.6).

A guided interview has proven to be extremely valuable in helping the FM practitioner determine the original source of the pain. Of course a patient could

TABLE 4.3 ■ Assessment Chart: Fractures, Operations, and Examinations

Traumas	Surgery	Examinations
Fracture, collarbone, right, 5 years	–	X-ray

A history of fracture of the collarbone, right side, 5 years ago is revealed.

BOX 4.6 ■ Abbreviations for Interview

SiPa = site of pain
Seg = segment
Loc = Location
Side = left, right, bilateral
lt = left
rt = right
bi = bilateral
const = constant
Rec = recurrent
VAS = visual analogue scale
d = day
w = week
m = month
y = year
ConcPa = concomitant pain
PrevPa = previous pain

have a local first-time trauma to an area with no previous history and only require local care. However, most complaints occur for no apparent reason although patients usually blame the last thing they did as the cause. Guided case histories are structured to gather the necessary information to decide which segments should be taken into consideration before starting the movement and palpatory verification procedures. Some patients have their own preconceived notions and may offer resistance during the interview. From the very beginning of the interview we must establish their trust and create an atmosphere where they feel free to tell us the story of their life. On the other hand, some clients are more than happy to talk and talk. For these kinds of patients the FM structural approach is extremely helpful in allowing us to promptly proceed to the next step.

Examples of Case Histories

A variety of interviews are described next dealing with the complaint of low back pain. Typical concerns of patients when they arrive are: "I have a back pain? Can you do something for it?" A complete history might reveal the answer. Four stories of back pain follow, and they may help us understand why there are no simple answers. All of these patients had the same complaint at first session: "My lower back is hurting me."

Patient 1 is a 30-year-old office worker. She has had bilateral low back pain for about 3 years (it comes and goes), but during the last 4 months her pain has increased for no apparent reason. The pain is more localized on the left side. Associated with her low back pain is an annoying disturbance posteriorly and laterally in her left pelvic and thigh area. Since she was in high school she has had more or less feelings of stiffness in her thoracic area between the scapulae. She had a horseback riding accident 4 years ago and hurt her left knee. (It is not bothering her at the moment.) Doctors investigating her lower back ordered a radiological examination that was negative (Table 4.4).

Patient 2 is a 45-year-old stay-at-home mother. She has given birth to four children without incidence. She has had severe bilateral low back pain for 3 years. It started when she lifted toys off the ground and felt pain on the lower and middle part of her back. A few days after the incident she felt referred pain in the left posterior part of her whole lower limb. Her physician ordered magnetic resonance imaging that revealed a disc prolapse at the L3/L4 level. At entry her main complaint was constant low back pain. Her left hamstring area tends to cramp during daily activities and she complains of left calf muscle pain during the night. In the thoracic area she complained of recurrent pain. Her right knee was traumatized 4 years ago but was presently asymptomatic (Table 4.5).

Patient 3 is an 18-year-old student who plays ice hockey and computer games and who complains of low back pain on his left side for 4 months. He states that it originated from a tackle in a hockey game. His pain is constant and increases with certain activities. A few days after being tackled he developed a stabbing pain in

TABLE 4.4 ■ **Case 1, Low Back Pain**

	Segment	Location	Side	History	Rec/ Const	Pain Modality	Notes
SiPa	LU	LA	bi, lt	Movement related, 4 months	Const	VAS 4/10	Worse when sitting, flexing, running
ConcPa	CX-GE	LA-RE	lt	?	Const	VAS 2/10	When LU worse
	TH	RE	bi		Rec	VAS 2/10	Sitting
PrevPa	GE	AN	lt	Trauma, 4 years	Not now	–	–

TABLE 4.5 ■ **Case 2, Low Back Pain**

	Segment	Location	Side	History	Rec/ Const	Pain Modality	Notes
SiPa	LU	RE	BE	Strain, 3 years	Const	VAS 5/10	Worse, sitting 20 minutes, walking 15 minutes
ConcPa	TH	RE	bi	Always	Const	VAS 1/10	Sitting
	PV-GE	LA-RE	lt	3 years, together with LU	Rec	VAS 1–3/10	Walking, night time
PrevPa	GE	ME	rt	Trauma	Not now	–	–

his left pelvic area. At present his low back pain is aggravated by rapid movements and turning in bed. One year ago during the hockey training season a minor strain in his left groin occurred. At present this area is symptom free (Table 4.6).

Patient 4 is a 35-year-old submission wrestler who works in a warehouse. He complains of low back pain during activities that encircle his back like a belt. The right lower back is a little worse than the left. Pain began while wrestling in a guard position where he was pulled and twisted by his opponent. His pain is constant and exacerbated when he is tries to lift something or rotate the trunk, especially on the right side. He also complains of pain in the left hip and thigh region. He thinks he might have sprained that area while wrestling possibly 2 years ago. Sitting more than 45 minutes seems to create pain in his thoracic area. He also

TABLE 4.6 ■ **Case 3, Low Back Pain**

#3	Segm	Loc	Side	History	Rec/ Const	Pain Modality	Notes
SiPa	LU	LA	lt	Trauma, 4 m	Const	VAS 3-6/ 10	Worse, sitting, extending, running, squating
ConcPa	PV	AN-LT	lt	After trauma, 4 m	Const	VAS 2/10 (move: 6)	All activity, special fast
PrevPa	CX	AN	lt	Sprain, 1 y	Not now	–	–

TABLE 4.7 ■ **Case 4, Low Back Pain**

	Segment	Location	Side	History	Rec/ Const	Pain Modality	Notes
SiPa	LU	RE	bi rt>lt	Trauma, 1 year	Const	VAS 2–8/10	Extension, lifting, rotating worse
ConcPa	GE-PE	RE-LA	lt	Trauma? Overuse, 2 years	Const	VAS 2–5/10	Worse after activity
	TH	RE	bi		Rec	VAS 1–2/ 10	Sitting
PrevPa	CL	LA	bi	Overuse	Not now	–	–

suffers from bilateral intermittent neck pain, which at the time of examination was asymptomatic. It has been bothering him intermittently for 2 years (Table 4.7).

The common complaint in these cases was low back pain. But in none of these cases was the pain specifically age-, sex-, work-, or sports-related. The associated painful activities did not determine the cause of the pain. The history can include traumas, injuries, sprains, overuse, misuse, or other things. Only a focused interview gives us a chance to get to the source of the pain. Even the complaint of pain in various areas of the back may not be significant regarding the underlying cause. Applying treatment only to the painful areas seldom solves the problem. Notice that in these cases there was some complaint of stiffness or other symptoms in segments either above or below the site of pain. These other areas may help to compensate for myofascial pain. They eventually may become problems on their own, resulting in dysfunction along a fascial chain causing pain, movement restriction, and changes in strength and coordination.

The answer to the question, "Why does my back hurt?" should be "It depends." It depends on personal history, previous problems, and other things that may have occurred. It depends on the body's reaction to previous stresses and the patient's capacity to compensate. Can we alleviate these types of problems? Of course we can. When asked this question, we can say that we do not know yet, but our job is to interview the patient long enough to understand their personal history and then locate myofascial dysfunction by movement and palpatory verification. First we locate the most symptomatic segments, sequences, or diagonals by case history and movement verification. Then we continue to find the location of the most symptomatic (densified) points, ie, CCs and CFs by palpatory verification. We combine treatment and functional testing to ensure that we are on the correct fascial plane.

MOVEMENT VERIFICATION (see Video 13)

The hypothesis determines the selected segments based on the history. The therapist then performs movement and palpatory verification comparing two to three of these segments to determine which of the 10 possible planes requires treatment. All of this information is put on the assessment chart to help the practitioner to determine the fascial plane to be treated. Movement verification (MOVE) is manifested in every movement direction, forward, backward, rotations, and side-bending (Fig. 4.32).

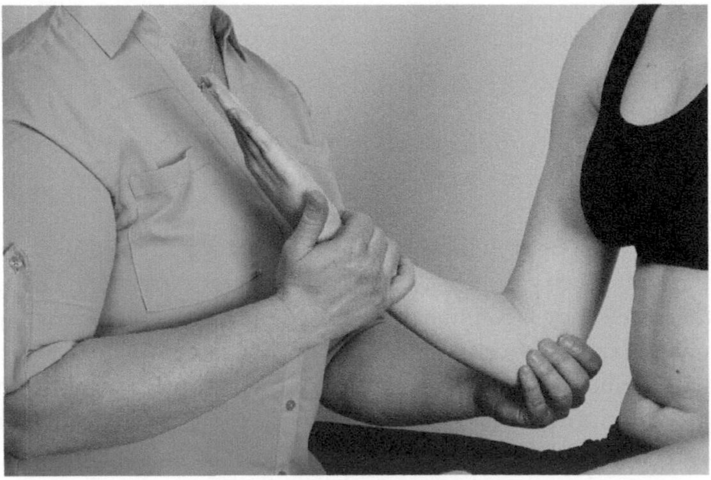

Fig. 4.32 Movement testing of the forearm, cubitus (CU) segment.

Movement tests of our body segments can reveal problems relating to that segment or side. They can reveal weakness, pain, imbalance, uncoordinated movements, deviations in the movement, poor balance, or recruitment patterns. It is important for the therapist to remember to test all movement directions to detect the problematic areas. This is also helpful for patients, because quite often they are complaining of pain and stiffness, but they are not aware of the imbalance, weakness, or other symptoms included in their complaint.

Movement verification tests are also very useful during treatment when a therapist is testing the effectiveness of the treatment (Box 4.7). This gives feedback to the therapist confirming that they are on the correct plane and allows the patient to follow the effects of the treatment. "I can now move more without pain. Movements are easier. I feel much more stable and stronger now." These are common

BOX 4.7

In fascial manipulation we use asterisks (*) to record the severity of the problem. * means a mild problem, mild pain, or restriction of movement or coordination. ** indicates more pain and more restriction on movement. *** shows severe pain, very restricted movements, and referral of pain to a centre of perception or other areas. Asterisks are an easy way to determine the most compromised sequences. There is no definite correlation between movement and palpatory verification, since all movements involve more than one plane. Therefore, treatment is focused according to the palpatory verification. Movement verification can be used more as an assessment tool, demonstrating the progression of treatment for both the patient and therapist (Fig. 4.33).

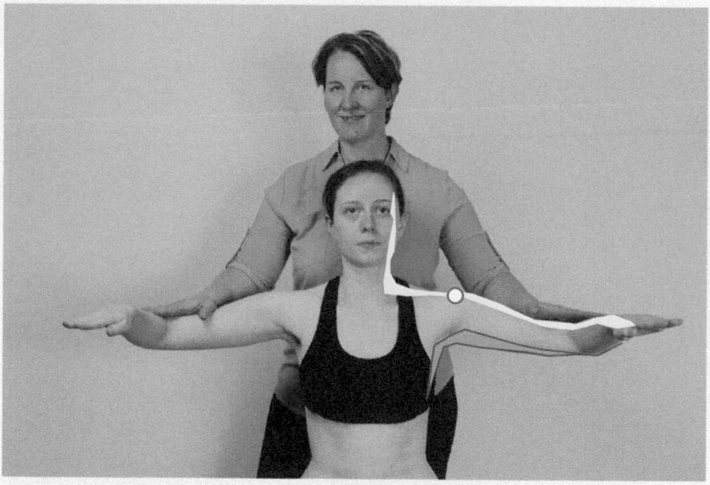

Fig. 4.33 Movement testing of the humerus (HU) segment. LA-HU reveals weakness. Yellow line indicates active sequence (agonist); blue line indicates balancing line (antagonist). Open circle indicates LA-HU centre of coordination.

statements after FM treatment. Patients are grateful to have an immediate response. This is highly motivating for the patient and the therapist. Quick results are mentally beneficial, reassuring the patient that their chronic problem can be eliminated, and life without pain or dysfunction is within reach.

The complete list of movement verification tests can be found in the text *Fascial Manipulation Practical Part* (Stecco and Stecco, 2009). The following movement tests are introduced as further examples. First we will concentrate on cranial points (CPs). CP1 points are located near the eye, CP2 includes the areas of the ear and jaw, and CP3 covers the points around the TMJ, jaw, and upper neck. The MFUs from the caput area can be tested by smiling and wrinkling the forehead, which tests the sagittal plane. Shifting the jaw from left to right and poking the tongue out and moving it from side to side will test the frontal plane. During these movements therapists should note deviations and asymmetry. Looking to the nose tip tests the horizontal plane. Pulling the apex of the ear downward and forward also tests the horizontal plane. The antagonist movement of ear pulling would be pushing back and down the tragus to tense the anterior auricularis muscle (Fig. 4.34).

The lower limbs can be affected by many traumas including ankle sprain or knee injuries. Problems can be ascending when they are affecting segments from distal to proximal (TA to LU) or they can be descending when the upper proximal segment (LU) is causing problems in the distal segment (CX). The hip (CX) segment may be impaired and altered due to previous ankle or knee problems or be related to previous or associated low back or pelvic problems. Sagittal plane testing of the CX can be tested when the patient is standing, by swinging the lower limb

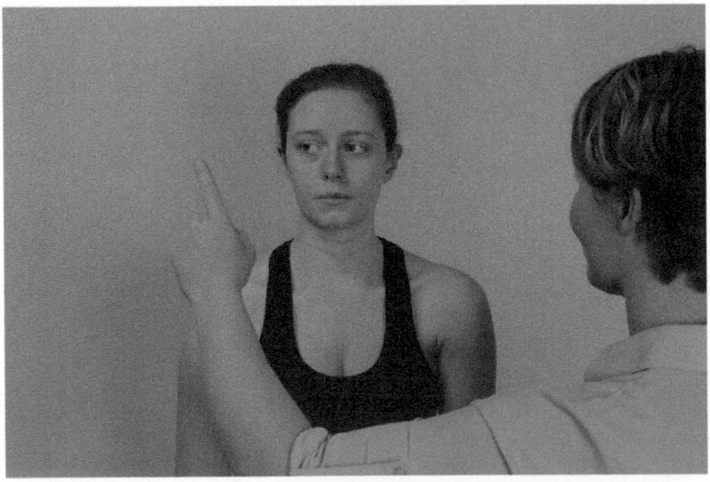

Fig. 4.34 Example of movement test of the head, CP1, segment. Patient is following the finger of the therapist with her eyes.

backward and forward. Antemotion movement in the sagittal plane can also be tested by resisted hip flexion in the supine position. Retromotion is tested with resisted hip extension with the patient prone or a high anterior or posterior kick from a standing position. Lateromotion (frontal plane) can be tested with hip abduction and mediomotion in adduction. These tests can also be tested with the patient supine resisting abduction or adduction. Extrarotation can be tested sitting where the patient lifts leg with ankle on top of the opposite knee and laterally rotating the hip. Horizontal plane for the intrarotation can also be tested from a sitting position as the patient is crossing one leg over the other (Fig. 4.35).

One example from the upper extremity is the elbow (CU) segment. This segment can become compromised often after a fracture of the forearm or wrist. It is a typical complaint of patients who work with a mouse or screwdriver. This is often due to an overuse problem or a patient doing something unusual such as painting the house or lifting heavy boxes. This segment is tested by using resisted movements to test for pain and/or weakness. The sagittal plane is tested toward flexion and extension both passively and against resistance. The CU frontal plane is tested by using isometric contraction with the extended elbow resisted against abduction to test for pain or weakness. For mediomotion the therapist will ask the patient to adduct the whole arm against resistance and verify medial stabilization

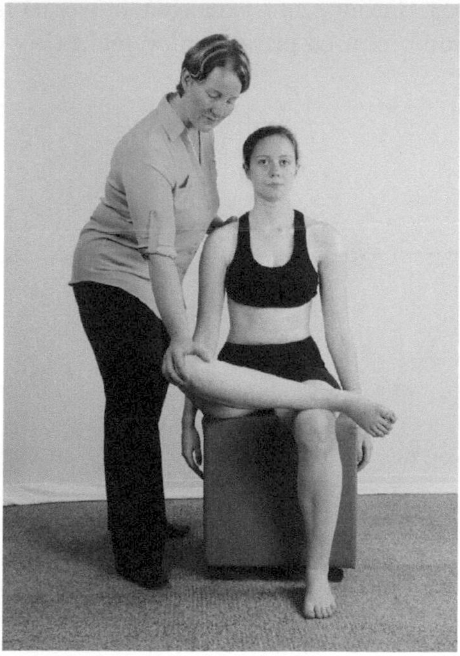

Fig. 4.35 **Example of movement test of the hip, CX, segment.** Patient is lifting the right side ankle on top of the left side knee and rotating hip outward.

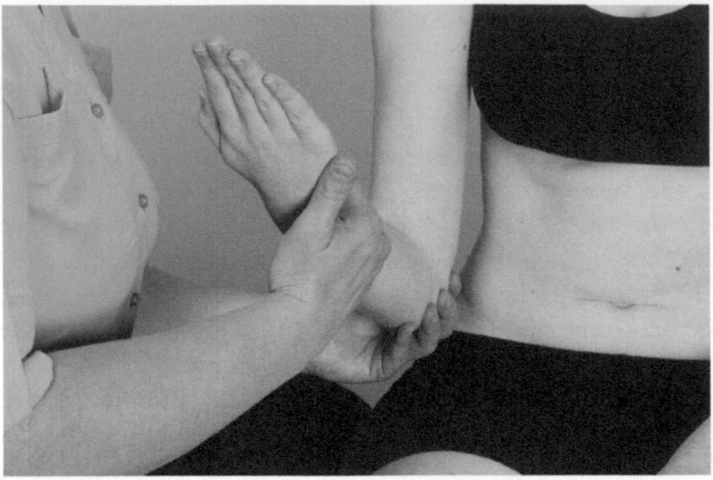

Fig. 4.36 Example of movement test of the forearm, CU, segment. Patient is flexing the elbow against resistance.

of the elbow. The horizontal plane can be tested by resisted supination and pronation of the forearm (Fig. 4.36).

All segments can be tested using active, passive, or resisted movements. Rotation, side-bending, flexion, and extension movements are basic tests to determine the most compromised plane of movement (Fig. 4.37).

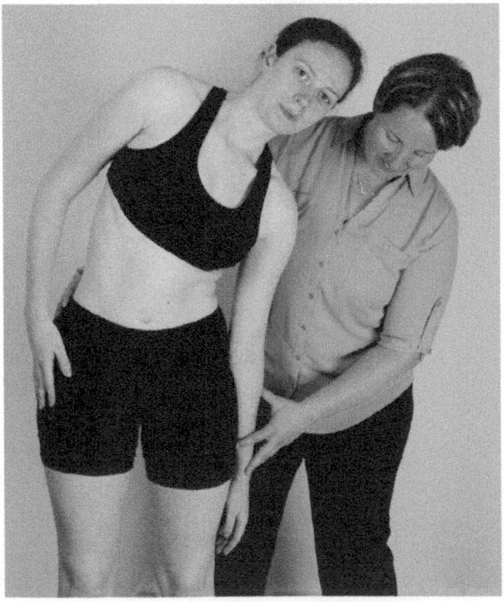

Fig. 4.37 Example of movement test of the lumbar, LU, segment. Patient is side-bending lumbar spine and the therapist is comparing sides.

CC movements are evaluated as above, along unilateral planes, while CF movements are evaluated along intermediate planes that involve a combination of movements. Examples are raising the shoulder 90° between the sagittal (anterior) and frontal (lateral) plane at 45° (AN-LA-HU) or standing and moving the hand inferiorly toward the heel by sliding the hand down the back of the thigh (RE-LA-LU). The presence of an altered CF is often associated with more complex and prolonged problems. Patients might be aware of some painful movement patterns such as getting into a car, which requires numerous available movements and it can stress many segments from the trunk to the lower limb. Skilful therapists can evaluate these kinds of movement patterns. Throwing is another example of a complex movement of the upper limb. This movement involves multiple segments and planes. An excellent time to observe a patient is the moment when she or he enters the clinic. How does the patient move, stand up, walk, and remove their clothing? Little hints may lead the therapist down the right track when choosing the segments for the movement verification.

PALPATORY VERIFICATION (see Video 14)

Palpatory verification (PAVE) is the most important part of the FM protocol. Every part of the protocol is there for a reason, but in this section the therapist is deciding the points that will require treatment in the chosen sequence. In this section both the knowledge and sense of the therapist are under magnification. Your fingers should be your eyes and ears, sensory devices that you can trust. What are we trying to feel in the tissue? The densification (Box 4.8). What is densification? It can be identified as a palpable thickening, ie, a dysfunction between the fascial layers. Loose connective tissue and its properties between the fascial layers are truly important and alterations in its properties are meaningful when we are palpating tissues. A therapist might feel a really crunchy area in

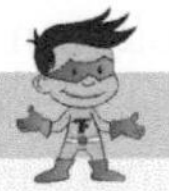

BOX 4.8 Densification

1. Palpable changes in the soft tissue—"crunchy".
2. Increased sensation of pain or tenderness, referral to distant areas.
3. Alteration of movement of fascial layers.
4. Alteration of joint range of motion causing pain and/or mechanical restriction.
5. Alteration of motor control—abnormal neural "input" and "output".
6. Alteration in force generation.

In fascial manipulation, asterisks (*) are also used to record palpation findings. * means mild pain and densification; ** indicates increased pain and densification; *** is a sign of severe pain, densification, and referred pain. *** points are designated as more significant. The sequence with the most asterisks is usually chosen for treatment, whether it's a sequence (centre of coordination), diagonal or spiral (centre of fusion), or combination of points.

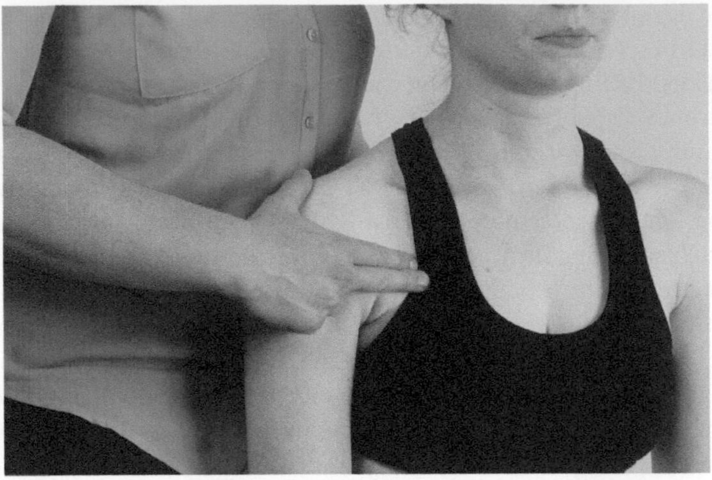

Fig. 4.38 **Example of palpatory verification manifested with fingers.** In this example, AN-SC centre of coordination is under the therapist's fingers.

the tissue or the altered tissue might feel larger, tenser, or restricted. A meaningful area is having a crunchy feeling that a therapist can identify. At the same time a patient might report sharp, deep pain, which may include referred pain. Movement between the fascial layers will feel impaired. This represents a densification or lack of tissue gliding that therapists can feel with their fingers. The patient usually can verify the findings of the therapist but sometimes there can be pain without densification. These points might be compensatory areas that do not require treatment (Fig. 4.38).

Dysfunction of the deep fascia can be due to modification of the viscoelasticity of the extracellular matrix (ECM). There is a misalignment of the endofascial collagen fibres, and this alters tissue capacity to elongate and adapt to stretch from the muscle. It means that that the density of the fascia has increased, thereby modifying the mechanical proprieties of fascia, without altering its general structure (Pavan et al., 2014). The ECM is like an ocean, and it includes many things. Hyaluronan (HA) in the EMC is thought to be one of its most important components when dealing with pain and dysfunction in the tissues. Hyaluronan affects ECM viscoelasticity and is responsible for creating a palpable difference in deep fascia. HA has many functions, one of which is providing a lubricant that allows normal gliding between fascial layers. Physical stress (trauma, overuse, postsurgery) changes the viscoelastic properties of connective tissue. The results of these changes will decrease the gliding potential of collagen fibres, resulting in an increase in overall tissue stiffness (change of liquid sol to gel) and possible pain. These changes of viscoelastic properties are palpable and are visible with

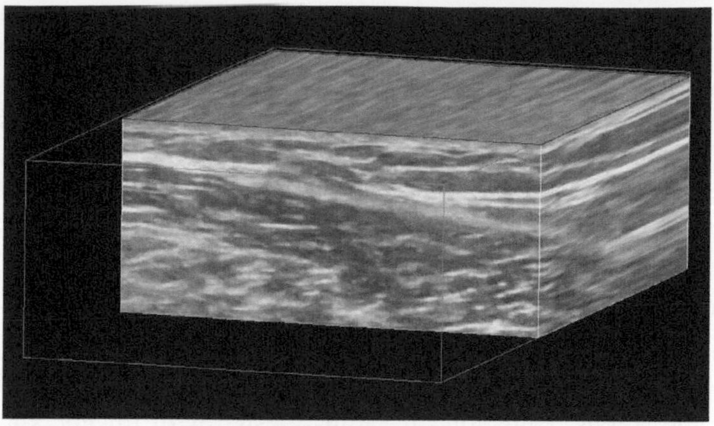

Fig. 4.39 Three-dimensional ultrasonography image of painful RE-GE point. *(Image courtesy of Jouko Heiskanen, MD.)*

ultrasonography imaging, especially with elastography (Luomala et al., 2014) (Fig. 4.39).

The FM therapist is attempting to find the worst points between at least two segments. After two segments are chosen, one method is to palpate all the points in one segment (six CCs and four CFs) to determine if one of those points is the most densified and tender. Then the therapist goes to the next segment and palpates all the points to see if there is a particular plane that correlates with the density of palpation of the first segment. It could be AN-TA (leg due to old ankle injury) and AN-CX (present complaint area). But what if another sequence (plane) feels similar? For example, LA-CX and LA-TA sequence also appear to be equally densified, too. In this case, in order to determine the involved sequence, the sagittal and frontal planes in a segment between the TA and CX, the knee (GE), points could be checked. In the knee the LA-GE could be normal and the AN-GE could exhibit the most density incriminating the anterior sequence as the "winner". In rare cases when two sequences feel like equal densities, the worst movement deficiency may be used to determine the plane to treat. In the above case we could not decide between the sagittal and frontal plane, but palpating anterior GE beyond doubt was the most painful, so one could decide to treat the anterior (AN) plane. Again in this case, after treating several of the AN points, was there a reduction in GE-AN pain? If so, you are probably on the correct sequence.

Palpation is really the chief method of diagnosis. When an FM practitioner is very familiar with point location, it is really easy to determine the chief densified plane, CC, CF, or spiral or even a combination of them. During palpation patients can report referred, deep pain, or other sensations. The therapist is concentrating on the state of the densification, the texture of the tissue, and the lack of gliding or sliding of the tissue. While patient response must be taken into consideration, the final decision is based on the amount of densification palpated by the therapist and not on the patient's response of tenderness or the most altered motion. Therapists should concentrate on feeling the densification, the texture of the tissue, and the movement sensation under their fingers. Comparing, sensing, and talking with the client are key elements in establishing a successful palpatory verification.

Examples of Segmental Palpation

We are now introducing only the CCs of a few segments. The *Fascial Manipulation Practical Part* (Stecco and Stecco, 2009) lists all CCs and the CFs along diagonals and spirals. Palpation can be manifested with fingers, knuckles, or elbows according to the segments. Palpation can be focused towards the superficial or deep area based on the problems that a patient is complaining about. Musculoskeletal disorders are most commonly palpated with deep friction, but swelling and numbness can be palpated more superficially using a broad contact.

Our first example is the head (caput, CP) points. This segment is palpated with fingers, because the points are located in small areas and the fascial layers are thin. Each plane in the head includes 3 subunits and all of those units are tested independently. CP1 points are often related to eye disturbances or headaches. CP2 is more associated with the ear and upper jaw problems, and CP3 relates to the upper neck or lower jaw problems like bruxism. All the CP points of the head can relate to the CCs and CFs of the neck and downward (Fig. 4.40). The neck area is extremely important when dealing with headaches, neck and shoulder pain, or movement dysfunction. In this segment the palpation is mostly performed with fingers. In the case of densification the transferred pain can be felt toward the head or shoulder girdle. Fascia of sternocleidomastoideus and scalenus area are important in cases of chronic neck pain, and this area should be balanced to maintain proper functioning of the neck (Fig. 4.41).

Lumbar pain is a common complaint (trunk area). It is recommended that palpation of this segment be performed with knuckles, because the mass of muscles is larger and areas of densification can be broader compared to the neck area. In this area CCs are located over the thoracolumbar fascia and abdominal sheath. Three-dimensional thinking is easy to understand in this segment. Tension in some parts of the fascial layers will alter the movement capacity and spread it distally, for example, to the lower limb (Fig. 4.42). In the lower limb we are studying the shin area or talus segment (TA). This segment is important, for example, after ankle sprains and it should be included in the palpation if the patient's history reveals some injuries or traumas targeted to the ankle or foot. It can be palpated with knuckles or elbows (Fig. 4.43).

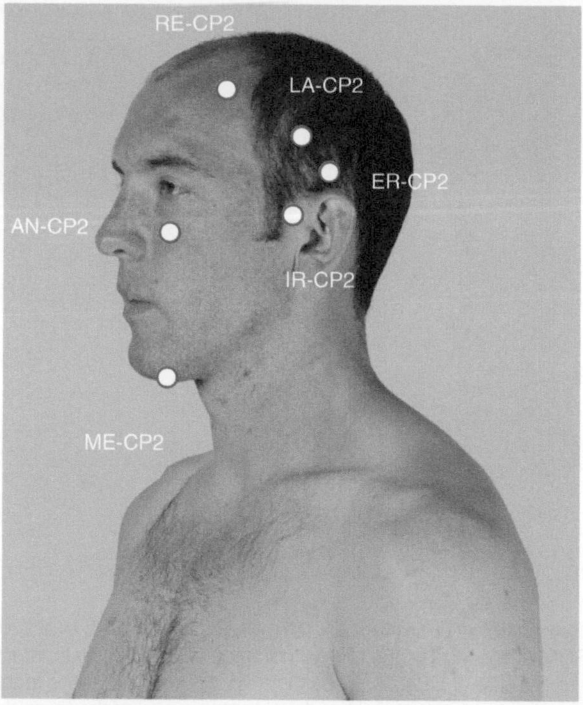

Fig. 4.40 Centre of coordination of CP2 segment. AN-CP2 is under the zygomatic process against the fibres of the zygomaticus muscle below the middle of the orbicularis oris. RE-CP2 is located over the medial eye where the forehead meets the frontalis muscle. Frontal plane point LA-CP2 is in the centre of the temporalis muscle. ME-CP2 is beneath the mandible, over the raphe of the mylohyoid muscle. The horizontal plane ER-CP2 is located above the helix of the ear, over the superior auricularis muscle, and IR-CP2 is anterior to the root of the helix, above the TMJ.

The elbow, cubitus (CU) segment serves as an example of upper limb segmental palpation. In this area myofascial expansions can be present in locations of CCs. Fascial expansions arising from the biceps brachii and brachialis connect to the antebrachial fascia. These areas are important when a patient is complaining of a tennis elbow or repetitive strain problems (Fig. 4.44).

Segmental palpation should include two or more segments to clarify the presence of dysfunction in a sequence or diagonal. This palpation protocol also includes concomitant or previous pain areas in order to locate and clear the areas that need to be treated. Although problems in movement may occur in some movement plane according to palpation, findings can differ. That is why we need to do careful segmental palpation to compare and analyse the state of the tissue. After recording the most densified and tender points in the assessment chart, the therapist decides which altered, diagonal, or spiral sequence to treat. Again, seeing and feeling with the fingers is crucial.

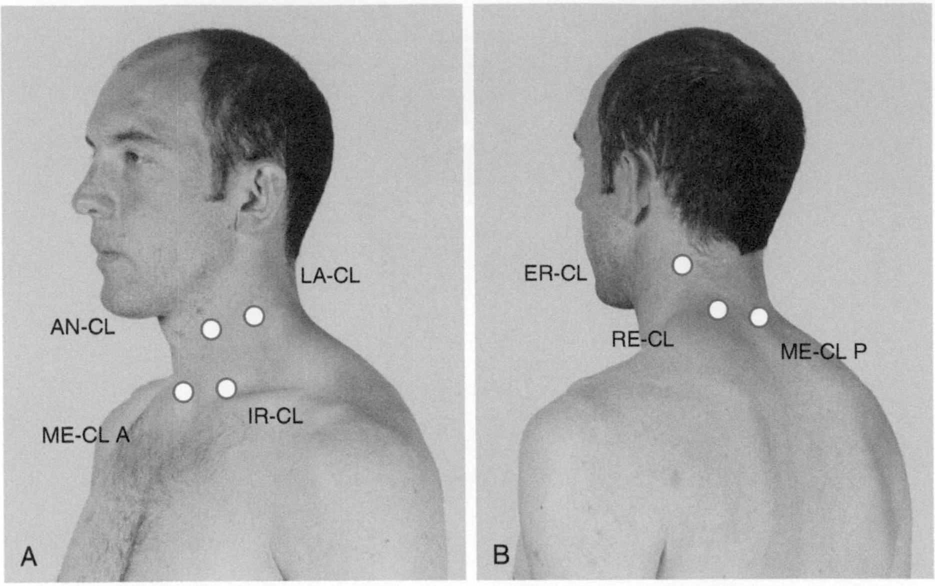

Fig. 4.41 Centre of coordination of CL segment. Sagittal plane point AN-CL is palpable from the anterior border of the SCM at the level of the thyroid cartilage and RE-CL is located over the mass of the erector spinae to the side of C5/C6. LA-CL point in the frontal plane is in the lateral border of the SCM, where the clavicular and sternal heads join, at the level of the thyroid cartilage. Anterior ME-CL lies in the suprasternal notch where the cervical linea alba travels. The posterior ME-CL is in the supraspinal ligament above and below C7. The horizontal plane ER-CL is anterior to the splenius, where the levator scapulae inserts onto transverse processes of C2 and C3. IR-CL is located between the clavicular and sternal heads of SCM.

FASCIAL MANIPULATION TREATMENT (see Video 15)

We must always respect the first dogma of medicine, which was stated by Hippocrates in 460 BC, *primum non nocere* (first, do no harm). The treatment should be applied with the least effort needed. FM treatment can at times be painful. Why? In the area of the CC where vectorial forces meet, there are tensions and increased viscosity in the fascial layers. Increased viscosity adversely affects many mechanisms in our body. Free nerve endings and other mechanoreceptors can be altered, creating pain. Mechanoreceptors, which constantly sense what is happening in our bodies, are compromised. The ECM between the fascial layers is altered due primarily to HA molecules that link proteins to the longer chains causing stiffer, painful tissue. Morning stiffness, loss of range of motion in different joints of our body, achiness, and pain when we overdo things are becoming more and more prevalent despite the worldwide exercise craze. There has not been over time any significant decrease in back pain or injuries.

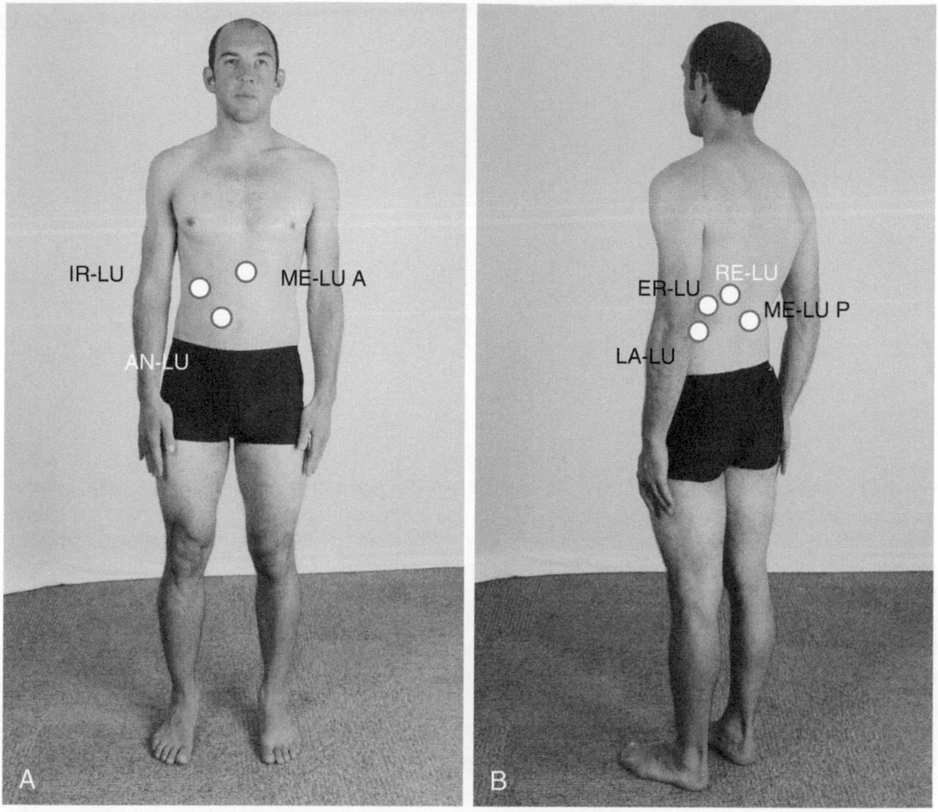

Fig. 4.42 **Centres of coordination (CCs) of LU segment.** AN-LU point lies over the rectus abdominis sheath at the level of the umbilicus. From the posterior side we can identify RE-LU over the mass of erector spinae to the side of L1/L2. Frontal plane includes LA-LU over the quadratus lumborum muscle, between the 12th rib and iliac crest. Mediomotion has anterior and posterior points. ME-LU a is palpable above the linea alba in three parts. First is below the xiphoid, next, halfway between the xiphoid and umbilicus, and last, over the umbilicus. The ME-LU posterior points are located over the supraspinous ligaments between L1 and L2 and L3 and L4. Horizontal plane has CCs of ER-LU located over the origin of the serratus posterior muscle, inferior from the posterior part of the 12th rib and IR-LU, which is on the edge of the 11th rib over the origin of the external oblique muscle.

There probably are universal fascial compensations occurring throughout the human and animal kingdom. This has been called the myofascial pain syndrome. FM offers a scientific and clinical plan to reverse the present-day situation (Box 4.9).

FM treatment often involves a special type of cross-friction massage to restore the normal properties of tensional points. When comparing tangential oscillation versus constant sliding, it seems that a more vertical pressure is more beneficial in

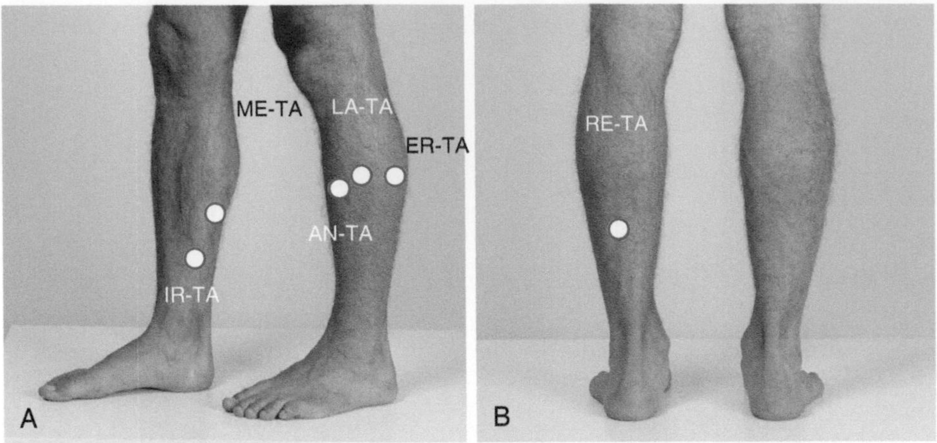

Fig. 4.43 Centres of coordination (CCs) of TA segment. AN-TA point is located over the tibialis anterior muscle belly between the ankle and knee. RE-TA lies at the myotendinous junction near the lateral head of the gastrocnemius. The frontal plane is palpated as LA-TA, over the extensor digitorum longus muscle, just anterior to the fibula near the middle third of the leg. ME-TA point is near the myotendinous junction in the lower leg where the soleus muscle merges with the medial head of the gastrocnemius. Horizontal plane CC of ER-TA can be identified behind the fibula over the fibularis muscle, slightly proximal to halfway on the lower leg. The intrarotation point IR-TA is over the tibialis posterior muscle, on the medial part of the deep interosseous fascia.

that it will help HA to flow near the edge of the fascial area under manipulation and this flow will enhance greater lubrication (Roman et al., 2013).

Increased temperature will return HA concentrations to a more sol-like substance. One of the effects of FM friction is to increase temperature. A possible reason why saunas or hot showers relieve pain is due to the changes that occur in the HA molecule. Reactions to FM treatments are variable. Initially patients may report sharp pain that rapidly decreases. According to Borgini et al. (2010), the mean time to halve the pain using FM is 3.24 minutes. But heat is not the only mechanism that alters tissue. Pihlman et al. (2014) found that 5 minutes of heating with ultrasound equipment did not result in a palpable response or decrease in pain sensitivity (VAS) statistically. This might indicate that while the heating properties of HA are important, combining it with mechanical load (cross friction) is necessary to solve the densification between the fascial layers. Dysfunction of gliding or shearing is usually due to changes in viscoelasticity as Langevin et al. (2011) and Luomala et al. (2014) showed. Changes in the viscoelasticity of loose connective tissue are visible with ultrasound, and these changes are palpable for the therapist and patient.

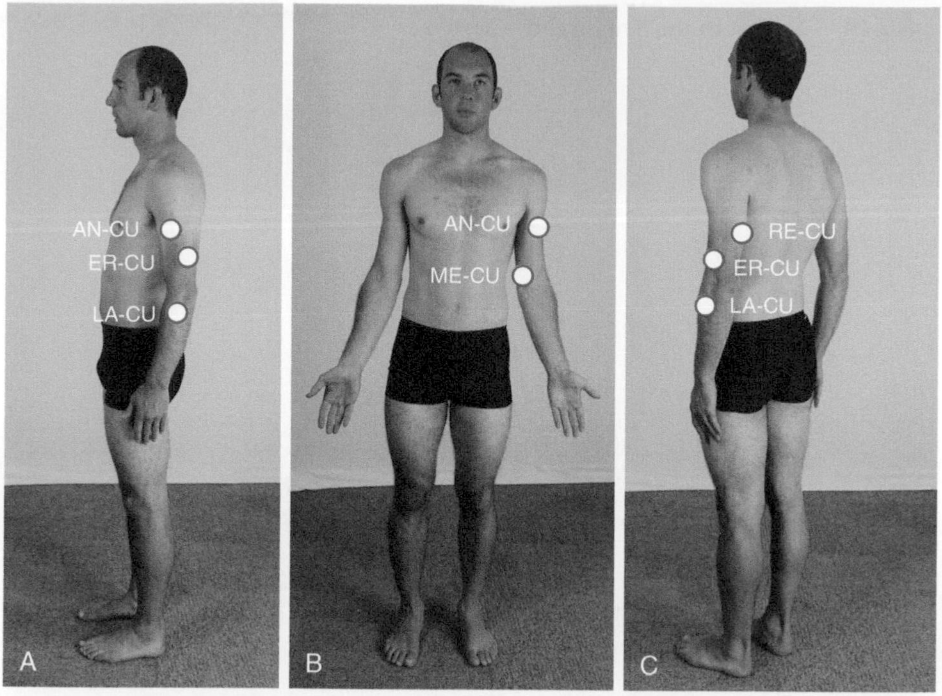

Fig. 4.44 Centres of coordination (CCs) of CU segment. AN-CU is located over the muscle belly of the biceps brachii, on the radial side of the muscle just below the level of the deltoid insertion. RE-CU is over the muscle belly of the triceps muscle, toward the septa that separates the medial and lateral heads and posterior to the deltoid insertion. LA-CU lies in the intermuscular septum just above the lateral condyle. The antagonist for LA-CU point is ME-CU over the medial intermuscular septum at the distal fourth of the upper arm. The horizontal plane covers ER-CU located over the origin of the supinator and brachioradialis from the lateral intermuscular septum over the triceps tendon and IR-CU over the pronator teres muscle below the elbow crease.

BOX 4.9 ■ Target of the Treatment

One of the prime goals of FM is to restore pain-free movement. It has been found that increased viscosity of our connective tissue fascia adversely affects proprioceptive feedback, muscle coordination, postural alignment, and muscle recruitment, and it is responsible for much musculoskeletal pain. Pain markedly diminishes when free nerve endings and mechanoreceptors are free to function normally (Stecco et al., 2013) (Fig. 4.45).

Continued

BOX 4.9 **Target of the Treatment—cont'd**

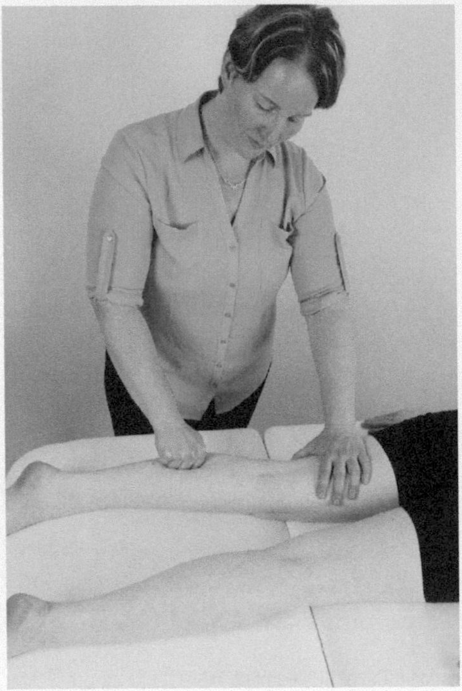

Fig. 4.45 Fascial manipulation treatment focused to the RE-TA point over the fascia of the lateral gastrocnemius muscle.

FM suggests different modalities of treatment based on the target tissue. If our purpose is to modify the superficial fascia, the treatment is usually performed with a larger hand surface. Freeing of the superficial fascia is necessary to stimulate the venous circulation and peripheral nerves. It also facilitates production and distribution of hormones that are fundamental for homeostasis of the body systems. Superficial FM is useful for treating internal dysfunction and in cases where the patient has excessive pain or where the whole fascial system is hypersensitive. For example, patients suffering with fibromyalgia or swelling will benefit from superficial FM. The superficial FM technique is also recommended at the beginning of treatment for children and animals. FM to the deep fascia is administered with fingers, knuckles, or elbows. Areas of treatment are fairly small, 1 cm to 2 cm. FM technique on CCs requires about 80% compression and 20% friction. CF pressure is about 60% compression and 40% friction since CF points are more superficial. In one treatment session approximately six to eight points are treated. Reducing fascial tension in one point is helpful in reducing tension in other points along the same sequence.

Reactions to treatment are varied. A patient can initially report sharp pain that rapidly diminishes. Referred symptoms are often immediately present, but they may also be absent or delayed. If after 4 minutes there is no change in the area you are treating, you might check closely in an adjoining spot (1 cm to 2 cm) or it is possible that you are not on a truly densified area. An alternative way of treatment is to avoid spending more than 3 continuous minutes on a point and treat points along the whole sequence going back and forth every 2 minutes. This will reduce the tension along the fascial chain, allowing the points to clear up sooner. Also if one point is particularly tender, it pays to treat above and below the painful area and return to it later when invariably its tenderness will be reduced. Treatment should be in the direction of the densified barrier. During treatment continue to "listen" to the patient and tissue. Both the therapist and patient are continually participating. The therapist will feel the changes in the tissue, the increase in gliding, and the softer feel all due to an increase in fluidity. If the patient complains that the treatment is too painful, reduce the compression or start the treatment from another meaningful point in the same sequence. Therapists are advised to use the least amount of compression to get the desired effect. It is also very important that the therapist maintain his/her own posture in a stable position with the least amount of stress. Fingers and wrists are an extension of a stable body, so keep your fingers and wrists relaxed by using your body to increase the amount of pressure (Fig. 4.46).

It is necessary to keep an accurate record of treated points on the assessment chart. Treated points and positive treatment outcomes are marked with plus signs (+ indicates minimal progress, ++ indicates medium results, and +++ indicates that the patient is free from pain and restrictions).

The FM therapist is aware that every visit should include a balancing of the sequence treated. Sequences, diagonals, and spirals work as agonist/antagonist

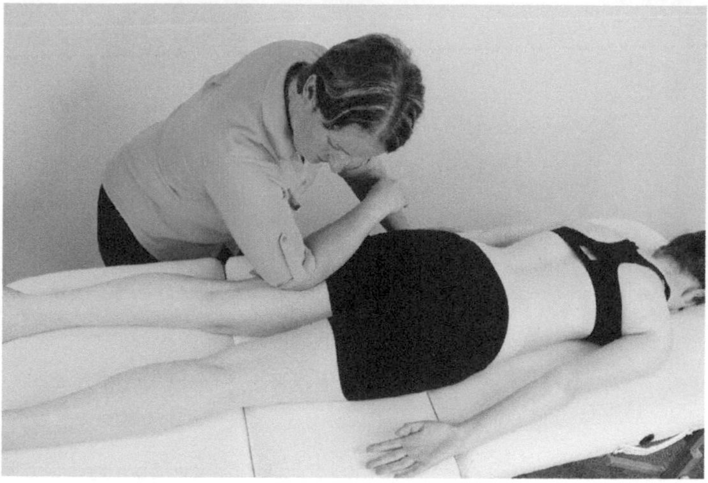

Fig. 4.46 **Treatment position of the therapist needs to be balanced.** Therapist uses body weight and keeps forearm and wrist relaxed.

pairs. If the therapist is treating antemotion, the balancing CCs will be in the retromotion sequence and vice versa. The same rules apply to the frontal and horizontal planes. It is recommended that only one sequence with its agonists and antagonists be treated per session. If more than one sequence is treated per visit it would be difficult to determine which sequence was responsible for either a positive or negative result (Fig. 4.47).

Treatment of the CFs that are related to intermediate movements are balanced between anteromedial and retrolateral and antelateral with retromedial diagonals. Spirals form complex networks and CCs from the horizontal plane can be added to these treatments since there are always rotational components to both spirals

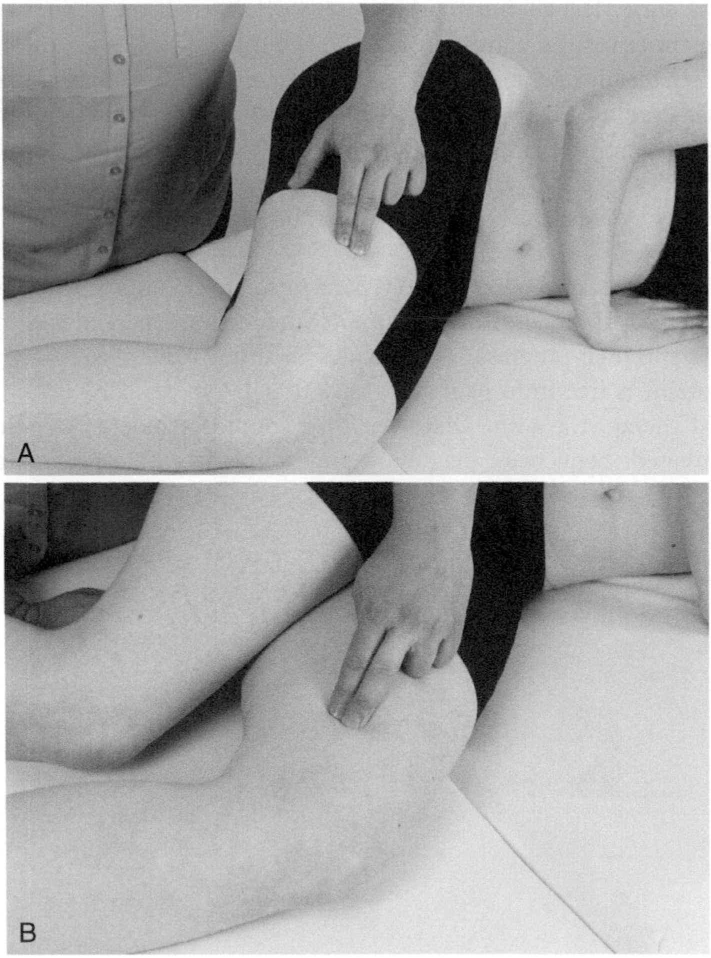

Fig. 4.47 **Idea of balancing the points.** Latero sequence point is balanced from the same limb from the antagonist sequence, in this case, mediomotion. Point to treat is chosen according to palpation and findings. Presence of densification should be noted. Also pain and referrals might be present.

and diagonals. These rules are present when dealing with musculoskeletal problems. After becoming proficient using FM with musculoskeletal problems, we can then decide to learn about the treatment of internal dysfunction. Part III in FM explores the relationship between fascia and internal organs. That world is revolutionary, consisting of combinations of CCs and CFs. With FM for internal dysfunction we can help people suffering from complex disorders and many functional problems. Quite often we have a mixture of problems arising from both musculoskeletal and internal dysfunction. FM thus becomes a total treatment alternative for many functional problems.

Sometimes a therapist might encounter problems due to the treatment itself. They may have used excessive pressure or applied too much friction (Fig. 4.48). During treatment it is necessary that the therapist remains completely focused on the contact and specifically over the density. If there is a continuous conversation going on with the patient, it is easy to move off the specific contact. Often a patient will report that you have moved from the point. It is acceptable to create a redness of the tissue, but there is never a reason to bruise an area. Therapists should maintain listening hands throughout the treatment.

Therapists should remind the patient that after the treatment there may be a painful reaction. The peak of the reaction is around 12 hours from the treatment session and the reaction will usually end after 48 hours. The reaction is actually beginning during treatment. It usually takes 15 minutes for the inflammatory

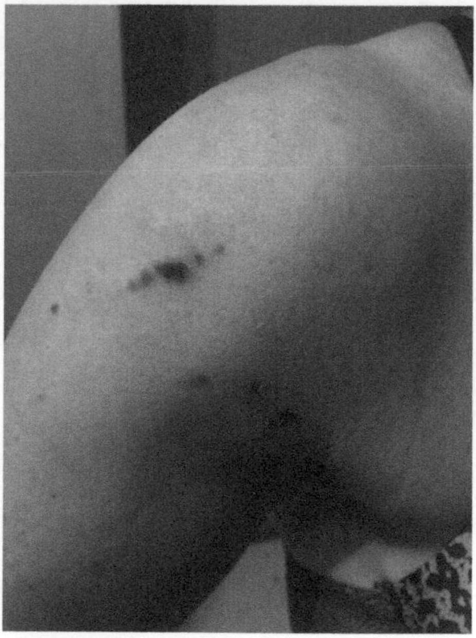

Fig. 4.48 Bruises are marks of excessive pressure or friction.

reaction to begin. It is important to inform the client so that they will understand why the next day they might experience soreness over the treated points. Other sensations are also common. Some reactions may be increased fatigue or even an increase in energy. In order for the inflammation to resolve and the fascia to become restored, the next treatment is scheduled about a week later.

AFTER FIRST TREATMENT: RESULTS, DECISIONS, AND PLANNING

Of course during each visit you continually re-evaluate movement and palpatory verification. The best case scenario is when the problem is solved in one visit, but quite often after the main problem is resolved additional information from the history is revealed. Children with their short history of symptoms are easier to treat, as are people who have suffered for only a short period and their problem usually originates from a singular event. Even when a patient reports very good results and no problems after the first treatment, depending on the history, it may be wise to schedule a follow-up visit in about a month and re-evaluate. Prolonged and long-term dysfunction and pain are cumulative and compensated for over the years and in these cases after one problem is eliminated another one eventually arises.

When patients return for the second treatment the therapist will ask three questions about their progress. Are they better, worse, or the same? If they report that they are better, then you most likely chose the correct sequence and will continue to evaluate and treat that sequence. If they are worse or if they felt relief and then the pain returned, it does not necessarily mean you treated the wrong sequence. There is a possibility that you did not adequately balance the sequence or even though a patient may complain, you discover on movement verification that their ranges of motion have improved and some tests are less painful. Maybe your treatment was not on an original causative segment and you just treated compensatory points. And of course you might have treated the wrong plane. Probably the worst news is that they feel no change. Again you will retest to determine if the patient's statement is accurate. If so, you may have to treat another sequence that was involved. It will be necessary to go back over their history since often at the second visit they remember an old injury that they forgot to tell you about (Table 4.8).

TABLE 4.8 ■ **Idea of Decisions**

The pain is increased	You may be treating the compensation; try the antagonist centre of coordination and palpate again
The pain disappears and then returns	Palpate again, change the plane if needed according to palpation
The pain is diminished, but not gone	Work in the same plane, palpate again further
No pain	Follow up if needed

CASE EXAMPLE

James, born 1965, spends his working day sitting behind a desk. He participates in activities such as yoga, Pilates, and cross-training. James has a problem in the right shoulder area. He has been visiting physiotherapists and they have prescribed exercises, but the shoulder pain persists. In fact, James remembers that his right shoulder has been tight even as a young boy at age 15. During the last 3 months the situation has been quite bad. His shoulder area is aching during the night and he has problems when training. He is unable to perform push-ups or chin-ups. The most pain is located at the anterior part of the shoulder joint.

He remembers that a few years ago he fell off a horse while he was holding the reins with his right hand. Since this event his shoulder pain has increasingly gotten worse. He was diagnosed with nerve root inflammation and received 4 months of sick leave. James has also had several operations. Fifteen years ago he was traumatically injured in a football match and fractured his right shinbone and the first phalanx of his right foot. James was thinking hard about his history and one big event popped into his mind. At 13 years of age while sprinting and jumping he felt a sharp pain in his left groin area. In his 30s he was operated on for a hernia in the same area (Table 4.9).

Treatment continues to movement verification (MOVE). After the interview during the first visit movement verification tests are performed to the shoulder

TABLE 4.9 ■ **James's Case History**

	Segment	Location	Side	History	Rec/ Const	Pain Modality	Notes
SiPa	HU	AN	rt	Movement related, 3 months (bothering him for 35 years, stiff)	Const	VAS 7/10	Cannot do push ups, chin ups. Night-time painful
ConcPa	HU-DI	LA	rt	Trauma, fell off horse, 3 years ago	Rec, 2 × a month	VAS 2/10	
PrevPa	PV	AN	lt	Trauma, 37 years	Not now		Hernia operated 20 years

Traumas	Surgery	Examinations
Football injury, 15 y ago, fract. Rt shinbone and I metatarsal	Operated: I metatarsal phalanx bone off from the right side big toe, rt shinbone operation	

TABLE 4.10 ■ **James's Movement Test Results**

Segment	Sagittal plane	Frontal plane	Horizontal plane
HU	–	LA-HU rt*	IR-HU rt***, ER-HU rt*
PV	AN-PV bi**, RE-PV bi*	LA-PV lt*	ER-PV lt*

joint (HU) and pelvic (PV) areas. Internal rotation (HU) was restricted with a limited range of motion. James also complained of a crunching sound in the shoulder joint. Movement of the pelvis was fairly stiff in anterior and posterior pelvic tilt. In James's case, sagittal and horizontal plane movements were more restricted than the frontal plane. Internal shoulder motion was the most painful of the tested movements (Table 4.10).

After movement verification in James' case, his right shoulder joint (HU segment) showed the most restriction. Palpation revealed that the horizontal plane was the most compromised. This part of the protocol is the moment where the therapist is verifying the findings and determining whether the hypothesis was correct. With palpatory verification, the points in the chosen segments, which are densified and showing the most asterisks in a particular sequence, are compared and affirm the sequence to be treated, in this case the horizontal plane. In James' case it was hypothesized that his right HU, SC, and PV were the segments that related to his problem. Therefore palpatory verification was performed on his right shoulder, scapula, and bilaterally in the pelvis. James' worst densifications were palpated bilaterally around the gluteus medius and minumus muscle (ER-PV bi and IR-PV bi). The points in the horizontal plane were not as severe in the shoulder (HU) area as in the pelvis but did correlate with the pelvic horizontal severe points. We therefore considered both segments involved. According to these findings, we decided to start the treatment from the area of the oldest injury, the pelvis. In this case, both movement verification and palpation verification agreed. Quite often this is not the case, as movement and palpatory verification might show different planes. When this occurs, the palpatory findings are considered more important in determining the treatment plane (Table 4.11).

Most of the time FM treatment can resolve 80% of the patient's symptoms if the correct sequence is treated. After treating a few points it is recommended that

TABLE 4.11 ■ **James' Palpatory Verification**

Segment	Sagittal plane	Frontal plane	Horizontal plane
HU	AN-HU rt**	LA-HU rt**	IR-HU rt*, ER-HU rt**
SC		ME-SC rt**	ER-SC rt*
PV	AN-PV bi**	LA-PV lt*	ER-PV lt***, ER-PV rt**, IR-PV bi**

the patient perform his or her most painful movement. If the therapist chose the correct sequence, there should be some reduction in the patient's complaint. Often we experience patients who leave our office without pain. These situations are of course most desirable for both therapist and patient. In the case of James, we had a great outcome after the first treatment. After treating the pelvic area the movement of the glenohumeral joint was normalized. He had a total pain-free range of motion. James said that he is now eagerly waiting to see if he will be able to sleep and train normally again. The next appointment was scheduled for 1 week later. It is recommended that for the next few days after treatment a patient's activities should be reduced, eliminating any maximum effort so that the body can create the optimal balance and homeostasis.

James was seen after 1 week. He was very happy with the results. Shoulder pain had resolved and he was now able to sleep through the night. He began to do pull-ups and chin-ups with no pain. He noticed after the first treatment that he had trouble coordinating his left leg when running. He stated that he felt unbalanced regarding lateral and medial movement as his foot struck the ground. He also noticed that the left leg was quite weak. In James' case the main shoulder problem was solved with one FM treatment, but an old problem became reactivated when the shoulder joint began to move freely.

James' second treatment session included testing of the gluteus medius on both sides. Testing confirmed that the left side was significantly weaker than the right side. With this information and after palpation we decided to treat points along a sequence that included the thoracic area, left hip, and pelvic area. After treatment his left gluteus medius strength test equalled the right side. James was rescheduled a month later and reported that he was no longer in pain and was able to train normally. His case was resolved in a couple of FM treatment sessions.

INDICATIONS AND CONTRAINDICATIONS

People often ask whether their problem can be solved with FM. FM represents a new paradigm in the evaluation and treatment of soft tissue. It provides us with a logical pathway of healing based on current knowledge. It allows us to understand the whole fascial system and its relationship to a patient's complaint. We are able to follow a path based on a patient's complete history to determine the original aetiology of their complaint. We are able to determine if we are on the right healing path and to change direction when necessary. By following FM procedures we are able to obtain excellent results.

Indications for treatment can be pain, tenderness, tightness, or problems in performing everyday tasks of life or sports. Diminished performance might be due to coordination problems, diminished force transmission, or reduced endurance. Many kinds of dysfunction can be improved with FM. Most musculoskeletal problems are indications for FM. Acute or chronic low back pain, tendinopathies, tennis elbow, shoulder pain, knee pain, headache, migraine, growth pain, etc., are typical complaints that we see. Skilful therapists applying FM can also help patients suffering with problems such as asthma, reflux, gastro-intestinal problems, PMS, speech dysfunctions, and dyslexia.

Some contraindications to treatment such as fever, infection, inflammation, and skin lesions should be considered. It is important to be aware of a patient's prescribed medication. If they are on anticoagulants, ask if they tend to bruise easily. Treatment may have to be administered with less tension. Are they on pain killers or anti-inflammatory medication? Drug therapy can alter the perception of the tissue preventing the patient from giving the therapist adequate feedback. With patients under heavy medications, an FM practitioner may have to consult with the patient's MD.

Precautions may be necessary when treating people with connective tissue disorders, such as Ehler–Danlos syndrome and HMS hypermobility syndrome. In these cases collagen synthesis is mutated and the connective tissue throughout the body becomes lax and hyperelastic. Skin, fascial layers, fasciae covering vessels, nerves, and internal organs are transformed. These people may benefit greatly from FM, but they will need a skilful therapist to apply the technique. This also applies to conditions such as haemophilia and diabetes. Cooperation with the medical profession is recommended. Acute injuries require precautions and often an FM practitioner can help the patient to cope better. FM treatment is often performed distant from the injury, thereby releasing the localized pain and altered sequence indirectly. For example after an ankle sprain we may be unable to treat points in the foot, but we can move higher in the lower leg like the talus or knee area. This may reduce oedema and release pain, allowing enhancement of the healing process.

Therapists have various tools to help the patient but the use of our fingers, knuckles, or elbows enables us to modify pressure and friction. FM can be performed on both the superficial or deep fascia. Layers of fascia have different functions and treatment is based on the fascial source of the problem. Only meaningful points, not compensatory points, should be treated. The next chapter will introduce case examples to highlight many situations when FM can be used.

References

Adler, S., Beckers, D., Buck, M., 2008. PNF in Practice, 3rd edition. Springer-Verlag Berlin Heidelberg, Germany.

Banks, K., Hengeveld, E., 2013. Maitland's Peripheral Manipulation. Elsevier.

Borgini, E., Stecco, A., Day, J.A., Stecco, C., 2010. How much time is required to modify a fascial fibrosis? J. Bodyw. Mov. Ther. 14 (4), 318–325.

Cyriax, J., 1984. Textbook of Orthopaedic Medicine. Part II—Treatment by Manipulation, Massage and Injection, 11th ed. Ballière-Tindall.

Kaltenborn, F.M., Evjenth, O., 2002. Manual Mobilization of the Joints: The Kaltenborn Method of Joint Examination and Treatment. Olaf Norlis Bokhandel, Norway.

Langevin, H., Fox, J.R., Koptiuch, C., Badger, G.J., Greenan-Naumann, A.C., Bouffard, N.A., et al., 2011. Reduced thoracolumbar fascia shear strain in human chronic low back pain. BMC Musculoskelet. Disord. 12, 203.

Luomala, T., Pihlman, M., Heiskanen, J., Stecco, C., 2014. J. Bodyw. Mov. Ther. 18 (3), 462–468.

Maitland, G.D., Hengeveld, E., Banks, K., English, K., 2001. Maitland's Vertebral Manipulation, 6th edition. Butterworth-Heinemann, Oxford.

Pavan, P., Stecco, A., Stern, R., Stecco, C., 2014. Painful connections: densification versus fibrosis of fascia. Curr. Pain Headache Rep. 18, 441. http://dx.doi.org/10.1007/s11916-014-0441-4.

Physiopedia, 2015. http://www.physio-pedia.com/Gait#cite_ref-Shi_6-0, 15.11.2015.

Pihlman, M., Luomala, T., 2014. Therapeutic ultrasound versus Fascial manipulation, differences in treatment effects. Conference book, association of fascial manipulation.

Roman, M., Chaudhry, H., Bukiet, B., Stecco, A., Findley, T.W., 2013. Mathematical analysis of the flow of hyaluronic acid around fascia during manual therapy motions. J. Am. Osteopath. Assoc. 113, 600–610. http://dx.doi.org/10.7556/jaoa.2013.021.

Shi, D., Wang, Y.B., Ai, Z.S., 2010. Effect of anterior cruciate ligament reconstruction on biomechanical features of knee level in walking: a meta analysis. Chin. Med. J. 123 (21), 3137–3142.

Stecco, L., 2004. Fascial Manipulation for Musculoskeletal Pain. Piccin.

Stecco, C., 2015. Functional Atlas of the Human Fascial System. Churchill Livingstone, Elsevier.

Stecco, L., Stecco, C., 2009. Fascial Manipulation Practical Part. Piccin.

Stecco, A., Gesi, M., Stecco, C., Stern, R., 2013. Fascial components of the myofascial pain syndrome. Curr. Pain Headache Rep. 17, 32.

Stecco, A., Macchi, V., Stecco, C., Porzionato, A., Ann, Day J., Delmas, V., et al., 2009. Anatomical study of myofascial continuity in the anterior region of the upper limb. J. Bodyw. Mov. Ther. 1 (1), 53–62.

Vaughan, C.L., 2003. Theories of bipedal walking: an odyssey. J. Biomech. 36 (4), 513–523.

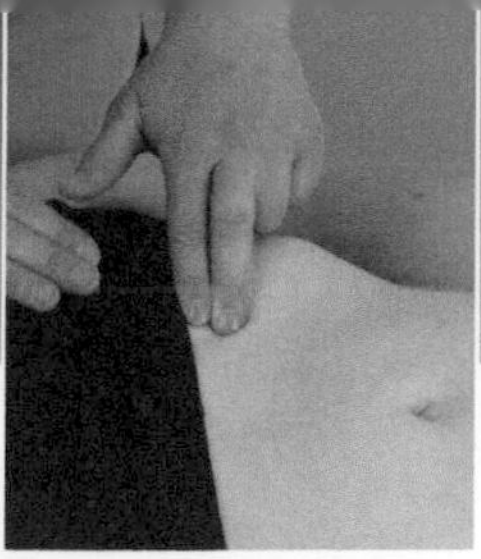

CHAPTER 5

What Kind of Disorders and Dysfunctions to Treat with Musculoskeletal Fascial Manipulation

Many common complaints of patients include musculoskeletal disorders such as back, knee, hip, or shoulder pain, stiffness, and loss of strength or coordination. Therapists face these problems every day and good decision-making and clinical reasoning will improve patients' lives. Treating these problems can also sharpen the therapist's skills with regard to the Fascial Manipulation (FM) protocol. FM protocol for musculoskeletal disorders is taught in level I and II. Patients often mention various types of problems and in level III of the FM protocol it is emphasized how internal dysfunctions are often causative of musculoskeletal disorders. Especially during the history-taking and treatment, it is important for the skilful therapist to be precise and keep the patient on the correct path. Too much irrelevant information can lead therapists on the wrong track when tracing the source of the problem (Stecco, 2004; Stecco L. and Stecco C., 2009; Stecco L. and Stecco C., 2014).

In this chapter we introduce some disorders and patient groups that will benefit from the FM method. The history-taking will support the decision-making, and movement and palpatory verification (PAVE) will lead the therapist to the right combination of points to treat. The case examples are real, but the names have been changed to protect the anonymity of the patients. Many other conditions can be treated with FM. Low back, knee, and neck pain and carpal tunnel syndrome are introduced. Children will also benefit from FM and treatment at an early age will help prevent future problems. Overall, FM treatment can be beneficial for various age groups and disorders.

Low Back Pain

Low back pain (LBP) is one of the most common musculoskeletal problems and the number one cause of disability worldwide. Approximately 70% of people will suffer from LBP at some point in their life. At this moment 1 in every 10 people suffer with LBP. The highest prevalence of LBP is in Western Europe, followed

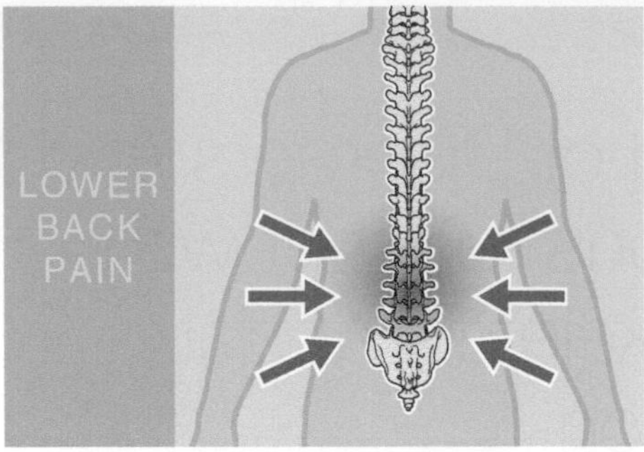

Fig. 5.1 The goal of the FM treatment is to help people move without pain.

by North Africa and the Middle East. The Caribbean and Latin America have the lowest numbers of LBP patients. It also seems that as the population ages, the risk of LBP increases (Hoy et al., 2014). It is evident that LBP strongly influences the world economically, individually, globally, mentally and physically. Many cases can be helped by FM treatment (Fig. 5.1).

Our modern society is based on sitting as we travel to work, watch television, and perform many sedentary daily activities. No wonder so many patients complain of pain in the pelvis or low back area. Langevin et al. (2011) showed the importance of gliding movement between fascial layers in the thoracolumbar area. Her study was designed to compare asymptomatic and symptomatic subjects. The research group hypothesized that people suffering from LBP had a reduced amount of fascial gliding in the thoracolumbar fascia. This indicates that loss of fascial gliding properties can be responsible for both pain and dysfunction in the myofascial system. Branchini et al. (2015) carried out a single-blinded, randomized, controlled trial using FM for chronic nonspecific LBP. The findings of this study support our goal in FM of establishing a pain-free and functional low back.

CASE STUDY 1

Michael is our example of a patient with LBP with a noncomplicated background. He is a 40-year-old man, who rides a bike, goes jogging (but cannot do it at the moment), and hunts. He works as a mechanic in a factory. He does not have any special medical condition or take any medication and his basic health is good. The only operation he had was the removal of his umbilicus 30 years ago.

Five years ago Michael was foresting and while moving frozen logs he felt pain bilaterally in his lower back. He received 2 weeks sick leave and painkillers. The LBP was relieved somewhat during sick leave and he returned to work. Every now and then he has been visiting a therapist who has been manipulating his lumbar spine. Results have been fairly good, but relief only lasts approximately 1 week. He has attempted to do exercises and stretching, but his back complaint still persists.

TABLE 5.1 ■ **Michael's Assessment Chart**

	Segment	Location	Side	History	Rec/ Const	Pain Modality	Notes
Si Pa	LU	RE	bi	5 years, trauma	Rec	VAS 4/10	Worse after sitting
Conc Pa	GE	AN	rt	Unknown	Rec	VAS 5/10	
Prev Pa	—						

Si Pa - site of pain; Conc Pa - concomittant pain; Prev Pa - previous pain; LU - lumbar area; GE - knee area; RE - located on the back side; AN - located on the front side; BI - bilaterally; RT - right side; VAS - visual analogy scale.

Two years ago he started to feel some discomfort in his right knee for no apparent reason. There was no accident, no injury, nothing! His knee was bothering him more and more and he visited a doctor. X-rays showed some arthritic changes in his knee. At present, his knee pain is recurrent and he is unable to run. He complains that his lower back is getting stiffer and feels similar to the LBP he complained about 5 years ago. Prolonged sitting and driving aggravates his back (Table 5.1).

Movement verification (MOVE) of the lumbar, hip, and knee areas showed restriction in hip extension and some discomfort in lateral rotation, worse on the right side. Lumbar forward bending was a little bit painful and lateral bending was stiff, especially when bending to the left. Palpatory verification of the fascial planes of the lumbar, hip, and knee areas revealed that the sagittal plane was the most involved regarding densification and sensitivity. Fasciae of rectus abdominis from the right side (AN-LU rt**), iliacus bilaterally (AN-PV bi***) and rectus femoris from the right side (AN-GE rt**) were all involved; Area of iliacus fascia (AN-PV) was extremely sensitive and densified on both sides, with some referral to the knee area. RE-GE rt** (hamstring area) was an involved antagonist from the right side. Some discomfort was also felt in LA-LU (quadratus lumborum fascial area) on the right side. Over erector spinae (RE-LU bi**) muscles, we could identify some alteration of fascial gliding. It was decided that the sagittal plane was the most compromised according to palpatory verification. Asterisks are indicating pain, densification and referrals. One * is marked if the point is painful or mildly densified. Two ** are marked if the point is painful and densified. Three *** are used when the point is referring somewhere and it is at the same time densified and painful.

Treatment was performed on points covering the area of iliacus fascia (AN-PV) on both sides, right lateral rectus femoris fascia (AN-GE), bilateral erector spinae fascia (RE-LU), and hamstring fascial area from the right side (RE-GE) (Fig. 5.2). Reassessment after FM treatment showed that the lumbar area was pain free, and range of motion, including hip extension, was normal.

Michael was instructed that on the day of treatment he should relax and the following day he could begin mild walking. Eventually he could start running for short

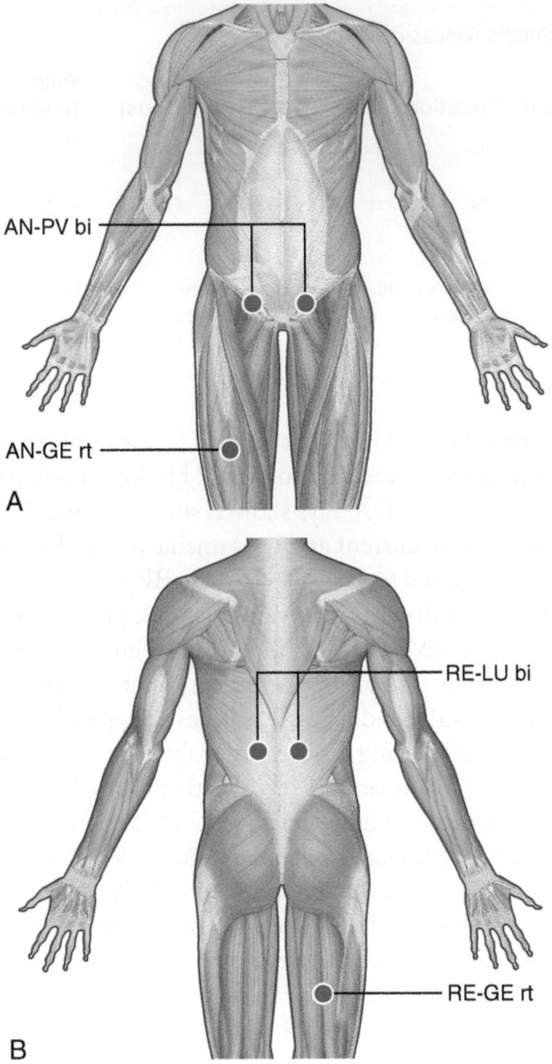

Fig. 5.2 Centre of coordinations (CCs) involved in Michael's FM treatment. (A) Frontal view. (B) Dorsal view. Fascia of rectus femoris from the right side (AN-GE rt); iliacus fascia and the area of inguinal ligament bilaterally (AN-PV bi); fascia of hamstring area from the right side (RE-GE rt); fascia of erector spinae bilaterally (RE-LU bi).

periods if his knees and lower back were pain free. He called 1 week after his first FM treatment and stated that he had started to run short distances and had experienced no pain in the knees or lower back. The next appointment was scheduled 1 month later. Outcome was excellent, as Michael has started jogging again and the LBP has not been bothering him since. Although when he came to the office 1 month later he had accidently sprained his shoulder area, but that is another story!

From this case we can highlight the centre of coordination of iliacus fascia over the inguinal ligament (CC of AN-PV), which is located over the iliacus muscle fascia medially and below to the anterior superior iliac spine (ASIS). In this area lies the inguinal ligament, which is often overlooked and rarely treated. This area is very important both anatomically and functionally because it is where the fascia of the trunk joins the lower leg. Myofascial force transmission from the thigh is transferred to the trunk and *vice versa*. In this area, thigh muscles attach to the inguinal ligament from below and all of the abdominal muscles attach from above. This was the key in resolving Michael's LBP.

Knee Pain

Knee pain is a problem that many of our patients are facing. Sometimes, however, it is just the tip of the iceberg. Knee pain could represent a compensatory pain for past injuries, trauma, or overuse spreading to proximal or distal areas. Finally, the knee is forced to overcompensate and pain results (Fig. 5.3).

CASE STUDY 2

Margot is a 38-year-old lady. She has been working as a secretary all her working career. She has one child, born in 2002. At the moment she has no time for hobbies and her only exercise is walking her dog. Pain in her right shoulder and left knee has been so bothersome that she does not have the motivation to attempt exercise. Her right glenohumeral joint was operated on in September 2014, after several years of pain. Bursectomy of the right shoulder did not relieve her pain. She does not remember the exact year the pain started nor does she remember any cause. At present her shoulder has diminished strength and restricted range of motion. Any type of shoulder exercise is painful. When Margot booked her appointment she complained mostly about her left knee, which has been bothering her for approximately 1 year.

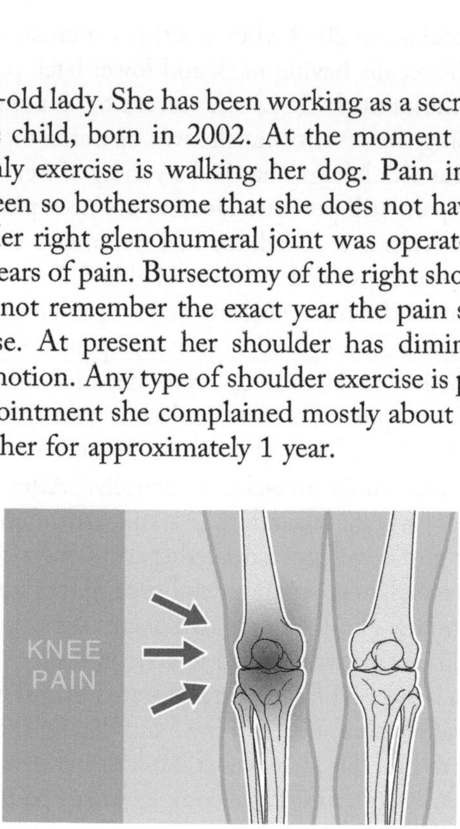

Fig. 5.3 Knee pain is often present due to dysfunctions of the lower limb.

TABLE 5.2 ■ **Margot's Assessment Chart**

	Segment	Location	Side	History	Rec/ Const	Pain Modality	Notes
Si Pa	GE	RE	lt	1year, trauma	Const	VAS 5/10	
Conc Pa	HU	LA	rt	More than 2 years, unknown	Const	VAS 3/10	
Prev Pa	CL, LU	LA	lt	6 years, trauma	Not now		

Traumas	Surgery	Examinations
Car accident, 6 years	Inguinal hernia, 37 years Bursectomy HU rt, 2 years	

Si Pa - site of pain; Conc Pa - concomittant pain; Prev Pa - previous pain; GE - knee area; HU - area of glenohumeral joint; CL - neck; LU - lumbar area; RE - located in the back side; LA - located in the lateral side; lt - left; rt - right; VAS - visual analogy scale.

She was in a car accident in 2009 when another car crushed the driver's side of her car. After that, she recalls having neck and lower back pain, but they are not bothering her at the moment. In 2012 she started to complain about heartburn. From the history-taking she recalls that she was operated on for an inguinal hernia when she was 1 year old. Margot has had a variety of treatments on her shoulder and knee but her pain still persists. Doctors are now planning to operate on her knee 2 months from her first scheduled FM treatment. Besides her knee pain, she complains of an overall general stiffness (Table 5.2).

Movement verification did not reveal any major problems in the knee area. Her shoulder joint had a reduced range of motion and pain on internal rotation. All other tests, both passive and resisted, were negative. Palpatory verification revealed primarily visceral points, so we decided to treat this case from a visceral (internal dysfunction) point of view. Treatment started on points on the medial side of the rectus abdominis muscles bilaterally. After treatment Margot expressed a feeling of overall relaxation. At this treatment session, points at the hip and shoulder girdle were also treated (part of the visceral FM approach) and the treatment was balanced at the sacral area. After treatment Margot felt much more relaxed and her shoulder pain had decreased. She still felt some tightness behind her left knee and we decided to schedule another treatment session 1 week later. At the second FM treatment she stated that she was able to ride her horse again. Her shoulder area was pain free, and during this period of time she did not have heartburn. Her left knee was still bothering her. It was slightly swollen and she had difficulty squatting. She complained of pain around the anterior part of the knee joint. This visit, both movement and palpatory verification revealed positive findings. Palpation revealed that the sagittal plane was the most

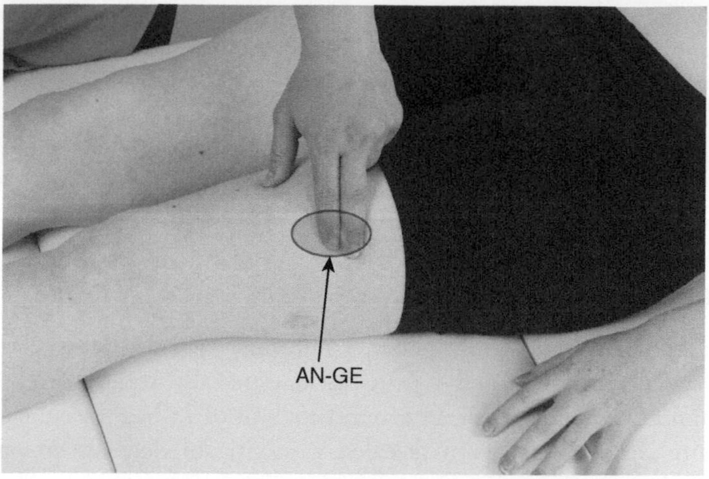

Fig. 5.4 Treatment of the rectus femoris fascia (AN-GE), centre of coordination.

compromised. We began treatment on the left AN-GE CC, which is located midway on the thigh between the vastus lateralis and rectus femoris muscles (Fig. 5.4). Along the same sequence we chose to treat the foot and shin areas and balance points (hip and knee) were treated on the retromotion sequence. These points were found on the left posterior hip and knee. After this FM treatment Margot is able to squat without pain. Margot's internal dysfunction was also related to her musculoskeletal problem.

In a pilot study, Pedrelli et al. (2009) treated a centre of coordination at AN-GE. This point is considered to be responsible for coordination of the quadratus femoris muscle and pain in the anterior part of the knee. This study was about evaluating a particular point rather than a particular sequence although it does add support to the treatment in this case.

After the second FM treatment session the next appointment was scheduled 2 weeks later. Although Margot felt much better after these two appointments, we still needed to verify the treatment to see if we could avoid the knee operation. When she arrived for the third FM treatment session it was obvious that she did not need an operation on the knee. She started jogging and riding again after years of being unable to do so and her knee was pain free. At the moment she feels some stiffness in her right shoulder area and after palpation it seems that the sagittal plane was also involved in the upper extremity. In the second treatment session we focused more on the lower limb and we checked the shoulder area. The third FM treatment included treatment of the sagittal plane concentrating on points in the neck, thorax, and shoulder. We asked Margot to call after 1 week to tell us how she was doing after the third treatment. Our conversation began with her saying that she had cancelled the scheduled knee operation. Now she has the energy to do exercises again, which will support her recovery.

In Margot's case, with FM we managed to improve her quality of life as she was able to start physical activities again, and we reduced her pain overall and restored her capacity for pain-free movement. Although her case was challenging, the outcome was good after following the FM protocol. Margot's background and previous accidents were compromising her body and altering her function. FM reveals its strength by following the guided protocol to determine the source of the pain and ultimately solve the case.

Neck Pain

Stecco et al. (2014) propose that patients suffering with chronic neck pain have thicker sternocleidomastoid and scalene fascia, especially in the surrounding area of loose connective tissue. Their ultrasound analysis of 25 healthy subjects and 28 patients with chronic neck pain revealed a significant decrease in pain and a decrease in loose connective tissue thickness after treatment sessions and follow-up. These findings support the hypothesis that the loose connective tissue inside the fasciae plays a significant role in the pathogenesis of chronic neck pain. The FM method is a perfect treatment tool for this kind of problem. The head works as a control unit for whole trunk. When we flex our neck and head, our lumbar spine will also flex and when we extend our neck and head, the rest of our spine will extend. The neck region is a meeting point for the trunk, head, and upper arms and because of that it is prone to become involved. Quite often when the neck is symptomatic it will affect the rest of the trunk (Fig. 5.5).

CASE STUDY 3

Paul is a 35-year-old engineer, who works on computers 8 hours per day. His hobbies are swimming and reading. He has been suffering with neck pain for the past 3 years. Onset of symptoms began when he fell on the ice during the winter and hurt his lower back and neck on the right side. Paul had some

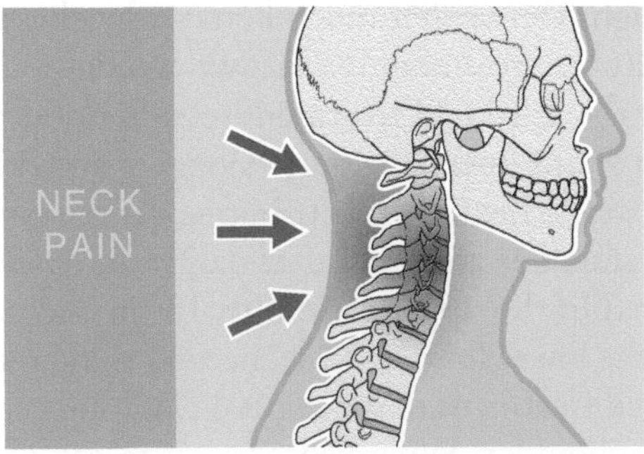

Fig. 5.5 The neck is the meeting point between the head, trunk and upper arms and the impairment of the fascial system of one of these parts can lead to neck pain.

TABLE 5.3 ■ **Paul's Assessment Chart**

	Segment	Location	Side	History	Rec/ Const	Pain Modality	Notes
Si Pa	CL	RE LA	rt	3 years, trauma	Rec	VAS 6/10	
Conc Pa	LU	RE LA	rt	3 years, trauma	Rec	VAS 2/10	
	SC	RE	rt	10 years, work-related	Rec	VAS 3/10	Worse when working with computer

Si Pa - site of pain; Conc Pa - concomittant pain; CL - neck; LU - lumbar area; SC - scapular area, shoulder girdle; RELA - located laterally and back side; RT - right side; VAS - visual analogy scale.

disturbances in his right scapular area before this accident. For approximately 10 years since he began working with computers he has felt intermittent stiffness and aching around his right scapula. He thinks this problem is because of excessive work and prolonged sitting. Swimming helps the scapular area, but during the last 4 months swimming has aggravated his neck and low back areas. Paul has no other history of accidents or operations (Table 5.3).

Based on his history and our hypothesis, we performed movement verification to the lumbar, scapular, and neck areas. His most compromised movement is on lateral bending of the neck and lumbar spine, especially to the left. The scapular area demonstrates restriction in the horizontal plane and weakness in lateromotion on the right side. Palpatory verification reveals the most densification in the horizontal plane points of the neck and scapula. After treating points located between the heads of the sternocleidomastoideus muscle bilaterally (IR-CL bi) and anterior to the splenius where the levator scapulae muscle inserts at C2, C3 on the left side (ER-CL lt), there was improvement in neck motion. The ER-SC point over the levator scapulae muscle belly was treated bilaterally and treatment was continued below the 12th rib over the external oblique muscle bilaterally (ER-LU bi). After treatment Paul felt much better and his range of movement in all directions of cervical and lumbar motion had greatly improved. He felt pain free and the next treatment session was scheduled for 1 month later.

Paul's case is a typical example of a musculoskeletal problem where distant segments are involved, ie, cervical and lumbar area (Fig. 5.6). The results in these cases demonstrate the value of using FM on the fascial kinetic chain. Restoration of fascial gliding properties enhances the body's capacity to move and rapidly reduces pain for our patients. These kinds of cases are gratifying to treat and the outcomes are rewarding for both patient and therapist. Restoration of fascial gliding potential will support the return to normal activities and hobbies.

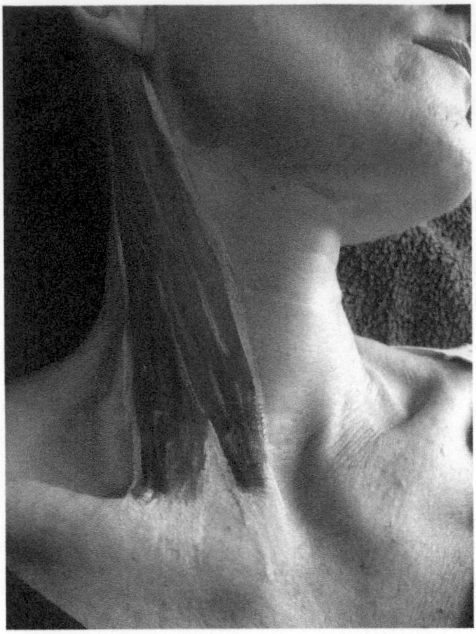

Fig. 5.6 Sternocleidomastoideus muscle painted on the neck, its fascial attachments are covering the whole neck area attaching to the other neck muscles, for example scalene and trapezius.

Carpal Tunnel Syndrome

Carpal tunnel syndrome is one of the most common nerve compression syndromes and responds to manual therapy. Architecture of the carpal tunnel consists of carpal bones, covered by the deeper transverse carpal ligament (TCL), and above the TCL, a superficial fascial reinforcement with its three layers that connect to the antebrachial fascia. The median nerve, together with the tendons of the flexor digitorum superficialis and profundus and flexor pollicis longus, pass through the carpal tunnel. The ulnar nerve passes over the same area but more superficially and medially in a tunnel called *Guyon's tunnel.* This tunnel is created by the pisiform bone and the superficial fascial reinforcement. The superficial fascial layers are a reinforcement of antebrachial fascia and work as a force transmitter to the longitudinal and lateral fibres. These structures are also related to spirals. The wrist retinaculum is well supplied with mechanoreceptors, including the proprioceptors. Centre of fusion (CF) points are located in this area and are responsible for the coordinative function of different myofascial units in the antebrachial area. The extensor retinaculum has direct continuity on the volar side with the antebrachial fascia. These structures enclose the wrist area and work as a sensory apparatus because of their rich innervation. The transverse carpal ligament is more likely working as a mechanical pulley and connects the hamate and pisiform to the scaphoid and trapezium. It creates the tunnel for the tendons (Stecco et al., 2010, Tang et al., 2012; Fig. 5.7).

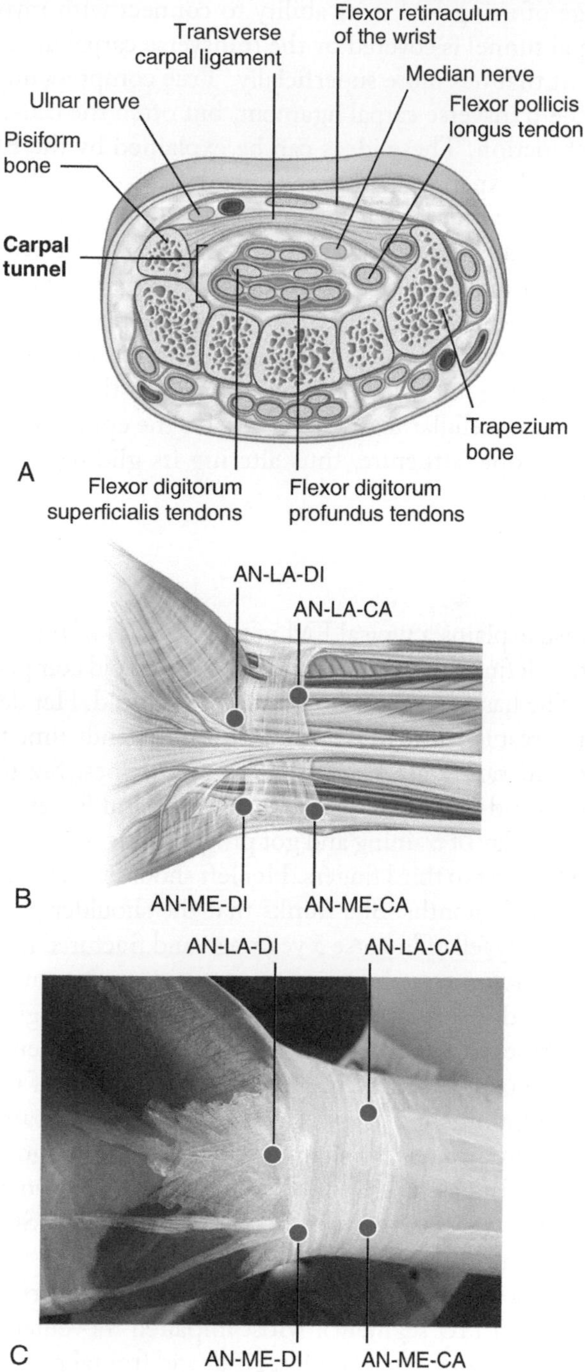

Fig. 5.7 Carpal tunnel and the centre of fusions (CF) in their anatomical locations. Points are located in the area of retinacula of the wrist. DI is indicating hand area and CA is marking forearm. AN-ME is indicating the line which is traveling to the anterior side of the forearm (ulnar side). AN-LA is located to the anterior side of the forearm (radial side).

The advantage of using FM is its ability to connect with myofascial kinetic chains. The carpal tunnel is covered by the transverse carpal ligament and a fascial reinforcement that lies more superficially. True compression of the median nerve is due to the transverse carpal ligament, but often the cause is more likely to be fascial dysfunction. These ideas can be explained by the FM protocol of sequences and fascial expansions from the pectoralis major to the biceps brachii, lacertus fibrosus, and antebrachial fascia. Dysfunction of this sequence might cause problems in some part of the sequence and mimic the symptoms known as carpal tunnel syndrome. Overuse or misuse of the wrist area can cause a transformation of the extracellular matrix of the deep fascia from a sol to a gel in multiple regions of the arm and forearm. This transformation might alter fascial adaptability and gliding and cause abnormal stress to the tissue. This increase of viscosity of the extracellular matrix may involve the epineurium of the medial nerve with its telescopic structure, thus altering its gliding properties (Stecco et al., 2009, 2013).

CASE STUDY 4

The following case explains a typical FM protocol. Parts of the assessment chart are added to better define this case. Wendy is a 40-year-old competitive rider who trains every day. She has one child who is now 10 years old. Her delivery was normal. Her chief interest in life is horse riding and she spends time teaching riders. Sitting, driving, and riding are her normal daily routines. Six months ago she started to have pins and needles in her left arm, wrist, and fingers. The symptoms occurred after a hard day of training and got progressively worse that evening. She felt numbness in the first to third fingers. Her left shoulder has been bothering her at night for the past 3 months. She thinks that the shoulder pain is originating from her wrist. Wendy fell off a horse 5 years ago and fractured her left collarbone (Table 5.4). It was not operated on and conservative treatment was inadequate. Sometimes she feels discomfort on both sides of her shoulder girdle, though not at this moment. Presently her left arm is extremely painful. Wendy describes the pain as more on the palmar side of the hand and flexor side of the forearm. She feels that every symptom she has is located in the anterior part, especially her shoulder and forearm area. She visited a doctor 1 month ago and he recommended a carpal tunnel operation based on electromyography (EMG) findings. Wendy first wants to try a manual therapy approach. She has an important competition coming up and would like to avoid surgery.

In the first treatment session movement verification was performed in the left shoulder area (SC and HU segment). Most impaired movements were internal and external rotation (horizontal plane); sagittal and frontal planes were pain free in both segments. Forearm (CA) segment revealed flexion with radial deviation of the wrist against resistance and internal rotation mildly painful. When testing

TABLE 5.4 ■ **Recordings After History Taken**

	Segment	Location	Side	History	Rec/ Const	Pain Modality	Notes
Si Pa	DI-CA	AN	lt	6 months, overuse	Const	VAS 8/10	Worse, night time
Conc Pa	HU	AN	lt	3 months, unknown	Rec	VAS 5/10	Worse, when riding
Prev Pa	SC	AN	lt	5 y, trauma	Not now		

Traumas	Surgery	Examinations
Fracture, collarbone, lt, 5 years	–	EMG, upper arm, lt, 1 month

Caput	Digiti	Pes
–	I–III, numbness	–

Si Pa - site of pain; Conc Pa - concomittant pain; Prev Pa - previous pain; DI - hand; CA - forearm; HU - glenohumeral area; SC - scapular area, shoulder girdle; AN - located in the anterior side; lt - left side; VAS - visual analogy scale.

fingers (DI segment), holding the claw position was painful and weak (horizontal plane). Wendy had also noticed this problem when riding and holding the reins. Resisted extension of the fingers also provoked mild discomfort and adducting fingers against resistance was weak. According to movement verification findings, the horizontal plane seemed to be the most altered.

After movement testing, palpation verification was performed in four segments: scapular, humeral, forearm and hand areas (SC, HU, CA, DI) and the most significant findings were on the sagittal plane. Points over the pectoralis minor (AN-SC) and lateral thenar eminence (AN-DI) caused radiating pain toward the left elbow. Left forearm (CA) segment was affected in every plane, but mildly. Also distally from the left shoulder (HU) segment all planes were impaired, but the most densification was in the sagittal plane. Points over the anterior part of the deltoideus (AN-HU) and infraspinatus fossa fascia (RE-HU) and the point between the brachioradialis and flexor carpi radialis (AN-CA) were planned to be treated from the left side together with the *** asterisks points of the left side AN-SC and AN-DI (Table 5.5).

The first treatment session began on the sagittal plane from the left side pectoralis minor area (AN-SC lt). Wendy says that when treating this point, she feels the referral in the lateral thenar area (AN-DI lt). This area was chosen to be treated next. After these points were treated, movement tests of the finger area (horizontal plane) were performed again. Wendy reported pain relief and improvement in strength. The antagonist side was balanced by treating the left infraspinatus

TABLE 5.5 ■ **Movement (MOVE) and palpatory (PAVE) verifications**

Move			
Segment	**Sagittal Plane**	**Frontal Plane**	**Horizontal Plane**
HU			IR-HU lt**, ER-HUlt*
CA	AN-CA lt*		IR-CA lt*
DI		ME-DI lt*	IR-DI lt**, ER-DI lt*
Pave			
Segment	**Sagittal Plane**	**Frontal Plane**	**Horizontal Plane**
SC	AN-SC lt***, RE-SC lt**		ER-SC bi*
HU	AN-HU lt**, RE-HU lt**	ME-HU lt**	IR-SC lt*
CA	AN-CA lt**	LA-CA lt*	IR-CA lt**
DI	AN-DI lt***		

HU - glenohumeral joint area; CA - forearm; DI - hand; lt - left; rt - right; bi - bilateral; SC - scapular area, shoulder girdle; HU - glenohumeral joint; CA - forearm; DI - hand.

RE-HU in the infraspinatus fossa, which felt densified and painful upon palpation. After releasing this point the forearm was checked. Densification still remained between the brachioradialis and flexor carpi radialis muscles (AN-CA) (Fig. 5.8). Treatment was finalized by checking antemotion and retromotion sequences for any remaining densification. Points over sternocleidomastoideus (AN-CL lt) and the erector spinae muscles lateral to C5 and C6 (RE-CL rt) were treated to create homeostasis for the upper body. Posttreatment movement testing (DI, CA, and HU segments) showed that all previously painful directions were now pain free.

The second treatment session was performed 1 week later. Wendy was feeling happy because her fingers and wrist had been pain free during the day, although she still felt some numbness during the night. She noticed that discomfort was present in the thorax and shoulder girdle area. Movement testing revealed that rotation of the thorax to the left was restricted. Some weakness was still present in the fingers, and palpation of the thorax, scapula, and forearm showed the presence of a spiral problem. In this treatment session the RE-ME spiral was treated from the left upper extremity and shoulder to the lumbar region. After treatment Wendy noticed improvement of thoracic rotation.

The third visit was scheduled 3 weeks later and when Wendy arrived at the office she had no problems in the upper arm. She was riding normally again and recalled that in the past she fell off her horse several times and had hit her head and left shoulder on the ground. This time movement tests were performed in the head and neck areas which showed deficiencies in the frontal plane. Palpation agreed with movement testing and treatment was performed in the head and shoulder areas according to the lateromotion sequence. In the left upper limb,

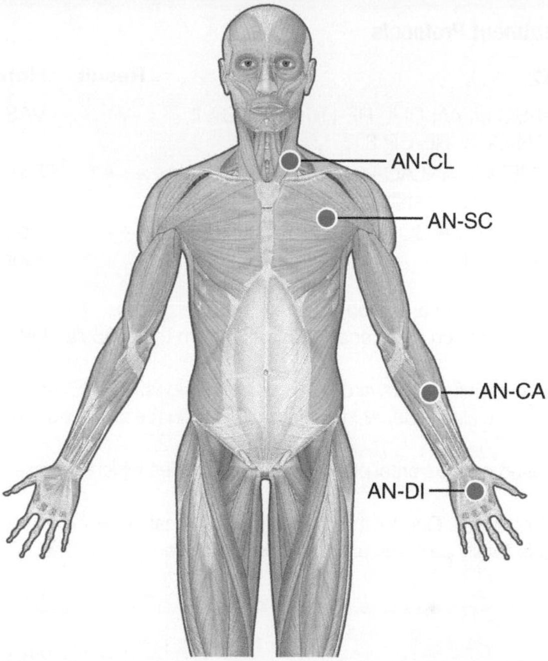

Fig. 5.8 Treatment of antemotion points in Wendy's case. AN-CL is located over the sternocleidomastoideus and its fascia, AN-SC is covering the fascia of the pectoralis major. AN-CA can be palpated in the middle of the forearm, antebrachial fascia. AN-DI is located in the palmar fascia.

palpation revealed densified points over the first dorsal interossei (LA-DI lt) and at the medial intermuscular septum, four fingers above the medial condyle (ME-CU lt). After this treatment (Table 5.6) Wendy no longer felt pain or paraesthesia. She was now ready to compete again with full confidence.

Pratelli et al. (2014) compared the effects of FM with laser therapy for carpal tunnel syndrome and the results were promising for manual therapy. The group of subjects who received FM had a greater reduction in pain perception and increased function after treatment. As in Wendy's case, the success of FM can be considered to be because of the attention paid to the myofascial continuity between the flexor carpi retinaculum, palmar aponeurosis, antebrachial, and brachial fascia. FM is a noninvasive way to approach this kind of disorder and in most cases the conservative model is enough to reduce symptoms caused by fascial dysfunctions. It seems that an alteration of the retinaculum is associated with fascial alterations along a sequence or a spiral, and in this way treatment of the fascia along the upper limb can improve the symptoms. Connections between the deep fascia of the upper limb and the epineurium of the median nerve can modify the telescopic structure of the nerve. FM is strongly recommended in these types of cases.

TABLE 5.6 ■ **Treatment Protocols**

Treatment	CC	Result	Notes
Treatment 1	AN-SC bi, AN-DI lt, RE-HU lt, AN-CA lt, AN-CL lt, RE-CP 3 rt	++	VAS 2/10
Treatment 2	REMEDI lt, ANLACA lt, REMECU lt, REMESC lt, ANLALU lt	+++	Pain-free after treatment
Treatment 3	LA-CP2 lt, LA-SC bi, LA-CP 3 rt, LA-DI lt, ME-CU lt	+++	No pain, no restriction or weakness

Points in the treatment session are given as an example.

First treatment session covered ante- and retromotion from the scapular, hand, forearm, humeral, neck and head areas.

Second treatment was manifested towards the centre of fusions. RE-ME line is covering the posterior side of the arm from the ulnar side. AN-LA line is traveling in the anterior side of the arm in the radial side.

Third treatment focused on the frontal plane, including muscles which are able to perform abduction and adduction.

Results can be marked with +. One + if the positive result is small. Two ++ if results are good and three +++ if the patient is totally pain free and there are no more dysfunctions.

Children in Treatment

Children can also suffer with many musculoskeletal disorders, such as headaches, shoulder pain, and "growth" pain. Traumatic events (eg, fractures, sprains, strains, and dislocations) may affect the myofascial system and alter the fascial gliding in children. Often children are undertreated, overlooked, and too easily medicated. Children react favourably to FM treatment. Therapists require "listening hands" and increased sensitivity, especially when treating children. The interview is sometimes tricky, because therapists have to consult the parents and matching their responses to the child's responses can be challenging. One advantage with children compared to adults is their shorter history. Most events and accidents are still fresh in memory of the family members. It is usually much quicker to reach a hypothesis and perform movement and palpatory assessment. It is often necessary to begin with a more superficial type of palpation before proceeding to a deeper level (Fig. 5.9).

CASE STUDY 5

Andy is a 6-year-old boy who serves as a good example. His mother is coming with him to the practice because he has been suffering with headaches since starting kindergarten. His kindergarten days are busy and the noises and hectic rhythm he is now exposed to seem to aggravate his symptoms. Sometimes he also complains of stomach pain, especially during night. These symptoms have been

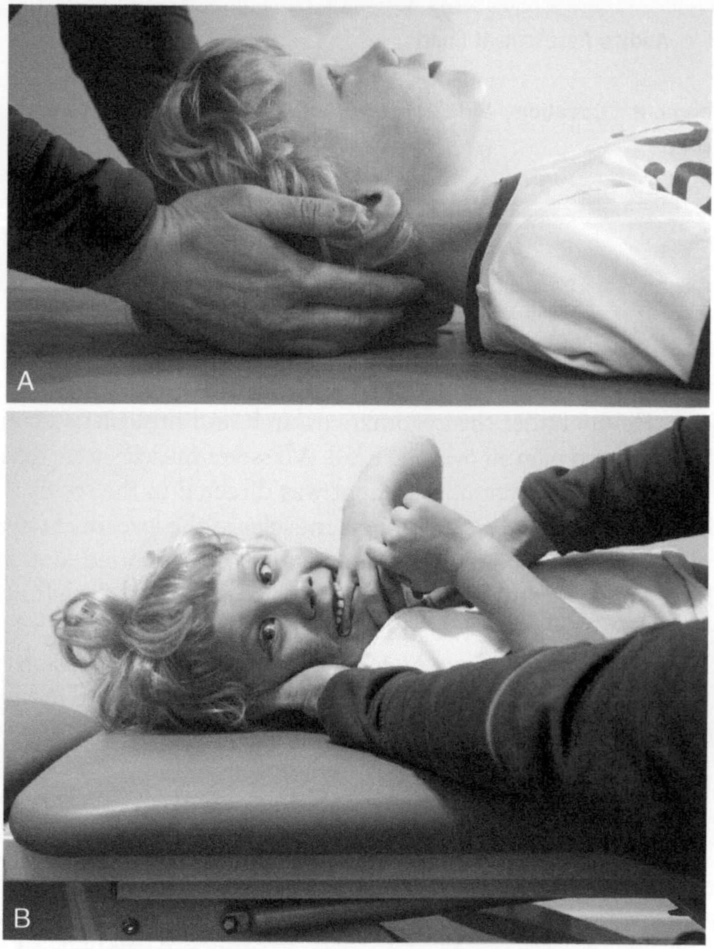

Figure 5.9 A child in FM treatment.

present for 5 months and they started when kindergarten started after the summer holiday. Otherwise he has been healthy with no history of surgery or trauma (Table 5.7).

Movement testing is done to the head, neck, and lumbar areas. Findings according to movement verification of the head revealed that the left eye is following moves towards lateral and oblique directions slower than the right eye. Movements of the jaw were restricted in lateral movements bilaterally. There were no movement verification findings in the neck or lumbar area. Palpation of the trunk on the rectus abdominis muscle was tender and densified bilaterally (AN-LU bi). The posterior side of the sternocleidomastoideus muscles was tight bilaterally and points over the erector spinae muscles lateral to c5/c6 (RE-CL bi) were

TABLE 5.7 ■ **Andy's Assessment Chart**

	Segment	Location	Side	History	Rec/ Const	Pain Modality	Notes
Si Pa	CP	LA	bi	5 months, overuse	Rec		Worse after days in kindergarten
Conc Pa	LU	AN	bi	5 months	Rec		Worse after days in kindergarten

Si Pa - site of pain; Conc Pa - concomittant pain; CP - head; LU - lumbar area; LA - located of the lateral side; AN - located of the anterior side; BI - bilaterally.

very sensitive. Points under the zygomaticus arch and orbicularis oculi muscles (AN-CP1 bi) referred pain all over the head. Masseter muscles were tensed, more on the left side. After palpation, treatment was directed to the rectus abdominis muscle bilaterally and to the erector spinae muscles at the level of c5/c6 and orbicularis oculi muscles also bilaterally (Fig. 5.10). Andy reported after treatment that he felt really tired. Movement tests were normalized and the left eye seemed to be brighter after treatment. His mother called a few weeks after the treatment and stated that his headaches were no longer present. On rare occasions when his headache returns Andy asks his mother to press points on his head in the evening. Otherwise he is doing fine.

CASE STUDY 6

The second case is Maria, a 5-year-old girl. She has had growth pain in her legs for 1 year. She started 2 years ago in a movement-oriented kindergarten where they walk a lot in the forests. Maria's pains started in the middle of the night and they have been more frequent the last couple of months. She wakes a few times per week because of pain and often subsequently limps in the morning and cries because of the pain. Her mother has given her medicine (NSAIDs) for the pain with good results and warm packs are also sometimes helpful, but the problem persists. She has no history of traumas in her life and she has been otherwise healthy (Table 5.8). Now her mother thinks that the medication may not be the best solution and she booked an FM appointment.

Maria did not reveal any pain or limitations on general movement assessment. Palpation of the trunk and ankles showed the presence of a dysfunction along the AN-LA spiral from the foot (PES) segment extending to the thorax. Treatment was started from the antelateral side of the foot followed by the retromedial side of the shin. The antelateral side of the knee was not densified, but the retromedial sides of the coxa and trunk were densified and sensitive. Maria is easy to treat and she is very responsive. Her mother is advised to call if problems continue or recur,

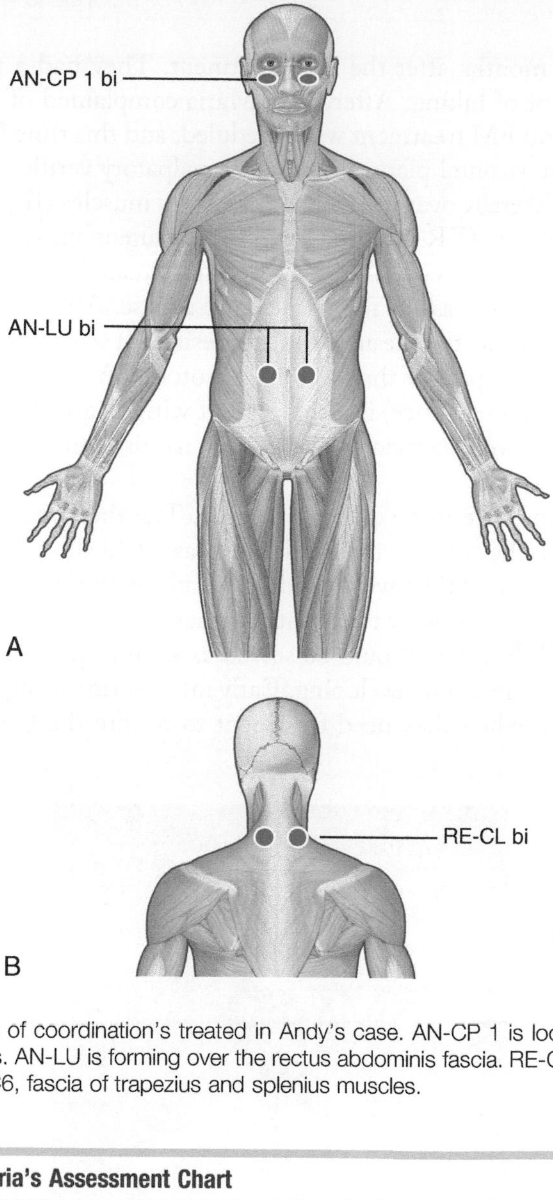

Figure 5.10 Centre of coordination's treated in Andy's case. AN-CP 1 is located in the inferior border of orbicularis. AN-LU is forming over the rectus abdominis fascia. RE-CL can be palpated in the level on C5-C6, fascia of trapezius and splenius muscles.

TABLE 5.8 ■ **Maria's Assessment Chart**

	Segment	Location	Side	History	Rec/ Const	Pain Modality	Notes
Si Pa	TA	LA/ME	bi	2 months, overuse	Rec		Worse at night time
Conc Pa							
Prev Pa							

Si Pa - site of pain; Conc Pa - concomittant pain; Prev Pa - previous pain; TA - shin area; LA/ME - located in the lateral and medial side.

and she called 2 months after the first treatment. They had a family camping weekend with a lot of hiking. Afterwards Maria complained of leg pain during the night. A second FM treatment was scheduled, and this time Maria had more problems in the horizontal plane according to palpatory verification. Treatment was performed bilaterally over the abductor halluces muscles (IR-PE bi) and over the piriformis muscles (ER-CX bi). Finally the gluteus muscle fascia near the highest point of the iliac crest (ER-PV bi) was also treated. Maria's reaction after treatment was promising as she felt relaxed and at ease. After this treatment session Maria has been able to hike and climb as desired. It seems that the horizontal plane was an essential part of the treatment protocol. As previously described a rotational (horizontal sequence) is often present with diagonals and spirals treatment. In this case, two treatment sessions were required to solve this myofascial dysfunction.

Children do not have to be difficult to treat. The therapist has to be able to communicate with the child on the child's level, as establishing a connection with a child is more important than with an adult. Results with FM treatment can usually be obtained in only one or two treatment sessions for the majority of cases. Dysfunctions and disorders should be solved as soon as possible to prevent the compensatory patterns from developing. Early intervention is important and children quickly learn when they need treatment to restore the homeostasis of the body (Fig. 5.11).

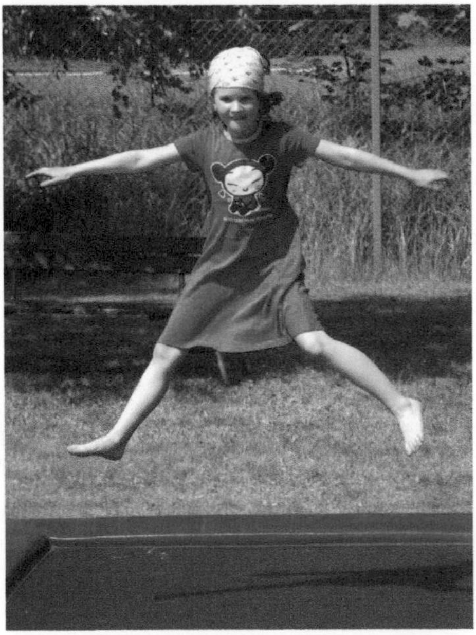

Figure 5.11 Children are being active after treatment and enhancing the effects of the FM by using their body.

Nowadays children with cerebral palsy, rheumatoid arthritis, scoliosis, and other congenital disorders may benefit from FM. While many neurological conditions cannot be cured, improving the peripheral nervous system by treatment of this vast fascial sensory organ may help children cope. Neurological rehabilitation may benefit from the FM method as a powerful tool to solve patients' myofascial problems. Ćosić et al. (2014) conducted a pilot study concerning postural hyperkyphosis. According to this pilot study it is suggested to combine FM with therapeutic exercises as a cost-effective approach. It was demonstrated at a 7-month follow-up that good results were obtained with a relatively brief period of FM treatment plus exercise.

References

Branchini, M., Lopopolo, F., Andreioli, E., et al. 2015. Fascial Manipulation® for chronic nonspecific low back pain: a single blinded randomized controlled trial. F1000Res, 4, 1208.

Ćosić, V., Day, J.A., Iogna, P., Stecco, A., 2014. Fascial Manipulation® method applied to pubescent postural hyperkyphosis: A pilot study. Journal of Bodywork & Movement Therapies. 18, 608–615.

Hoy, D., March, L., Brooks, P., Blyth, F., Woolf, A., Bain, C., et al., 2014. The global burden of low back pain: estimates from the Global Burden of Disease 2010 study. Ann. Rheum. Dis. http://dx.doi.org/10.1136/annrheumdis-2013-204428, published online 24 March 2014.

Langevin, H., Fox, J.R., Koptiuch, C., Badger, G.J., Greenan-Naumann, A.C., Bouffard, N.A., et al., 2011. Reduced thoracolumbar fascia shear strain in human chronic low back pain. BMC Musculoskelet. Disord. http://dx.doi.org/10.1186/1471-2474-12-203.

Pedrelli, A., Stecco, C., Day, J.A., 2009. Treating patellar tendinopathy with fascial manipulation. J. Bodyw. Mov. Ther. 13, 73–80.

Pratelli, E., Pintucci, M., Cultrera, P., Baldini, E., Stecco, A., Petroncelli, A., et al., 2014. Conservative treatment of carpal tunnel syndrome: comparison between laser therapy and fascial manipulation. J. Bodyw. Mov. Ther. http://dx.doi.org/10.1016/j.jbmt.2014.08.002.

Stecco, L., 2004. Fascial Manipulation for Musculoskeletal Pain. Piccin, Padua, Italy.

Stecco, L., Stecco, C., 2009. Fascial Manipulation Practical Part. Piccin, Padua, Italy.

Stecco, A., Macchi, V., Stecco, C., Porzionato, A., Ann Day, J., Delmas, V., et al., 2009. Anatomical study of myofascial continuity in the anterior region of the upper limb. J. Bodyw. Mov. Ther. 13 (1), 53–62.

Stecco, C., Macchi, V., Lancerotto, L., Tiengo, C., Porzionato, A., De Caro, R., 2010. Comparison of transverse carpal ligament and flexor retinaculum terminology for the wrist. J. Hand Surg. 35, 746–753. http://dx.doi.org/10.1016/j.jhsa.2010.01.031.

Stecco, A., Gesi, M., Stecco, C., Stern, R., 2013. Fascial components of the myofascial pain syndrome. Curr. Pain Headache Rep. 17, 32.

Stecco, A., Meneghini, A., Stern, R., Stecco, C., Imamura, M., 2014. Ultrasonography in myofascial neck pain: randomized clinical trial for diagnosis and follow-up. Surg. Radiol. Anat. 36 (3), 243–253.

Stecco, L., Stecco, C., 2014. Fascial Manipulation for Internal Dysfunction. Piccin, Padua, Italy.

Tang, J.B., Amadio, P.C., Guimberteau, J.C., Chang, J., 2012. Tendon Surgery of the Hand. Elsevier. pp 3–16.

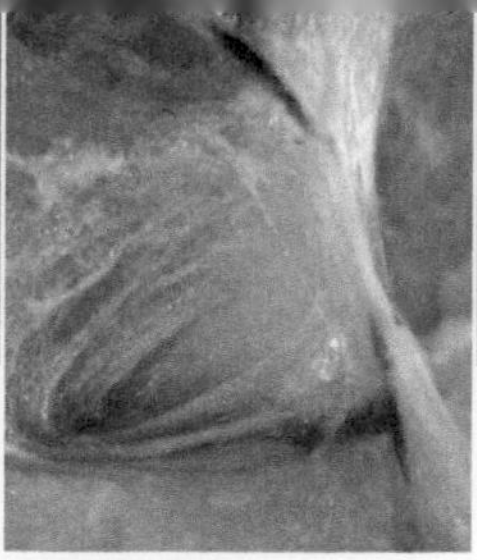

CHAPTER 6

Fascial Manipulation for Internal Dysfunctions

A therapist using fascial manipulation (FM) would definitely think about FM for internal dysfunctions (FMID) when symptoms of a musculoskeletal problem are not relieved or reappear soon after treatment. Upon examination, these patients do not complain of pain on movement verification (MOVE). Their pain is diffuse, poorly defined, and fluctuating in onset. Their history will also reveal internal dysfunction with symptoms relating, for example, to their digestive, glandular, or respiratory system. FMID is aimed at treating functional internal disturbances rather than actual pathology. Luigi Stecco wrote a textbook (Stecco and Stecco, 2014) reinforcing the idea of a fascial therapeutic approach to internal dysfunction by recognizing, for example, the close relationship between the internal fasciae and the autonomic nervous system. These kinds of missing links reveal the global relationship of the human fascial system and support the concept that the myofascial system is closely related to the internal system.

Internal Fasciae

A principal function of the internal fascia is to ensure the autonomy of the organs and viscera with respect to the musculoskeletal system (ie, the abdominal wall). It also supports and maintains the position and movement of the viscera and organs. The internal fasciae participate in managing and coordinating an organ's motility and mobility. The inner fasciae also ensure proper passage for vessels, nerves, and lymphatic vessels. FMID administers friction and pressure to the wall of the trunk to correct the overall tension of the body. Correcting abdominal surface tension affects the deeper fascia, thereby restoring the mobility and function of organs.

Based on dissection findings we can divide the abdominal internal fasciae into investing and insertional fasciae (Fig. 6.1). Investing fasciae are adherent to the organ, vessel, or gland and have an important role in local coordination. In this way investing fasciae give form to the organ. They are very sensitive to stretching stimuli and their autonomic innervation gives them local coordinative properties. Investing fasciae can be compared to epimysium, which is a similar structure in the musculoskeletal system. Investing fascia of the organs is thin, elastic, and

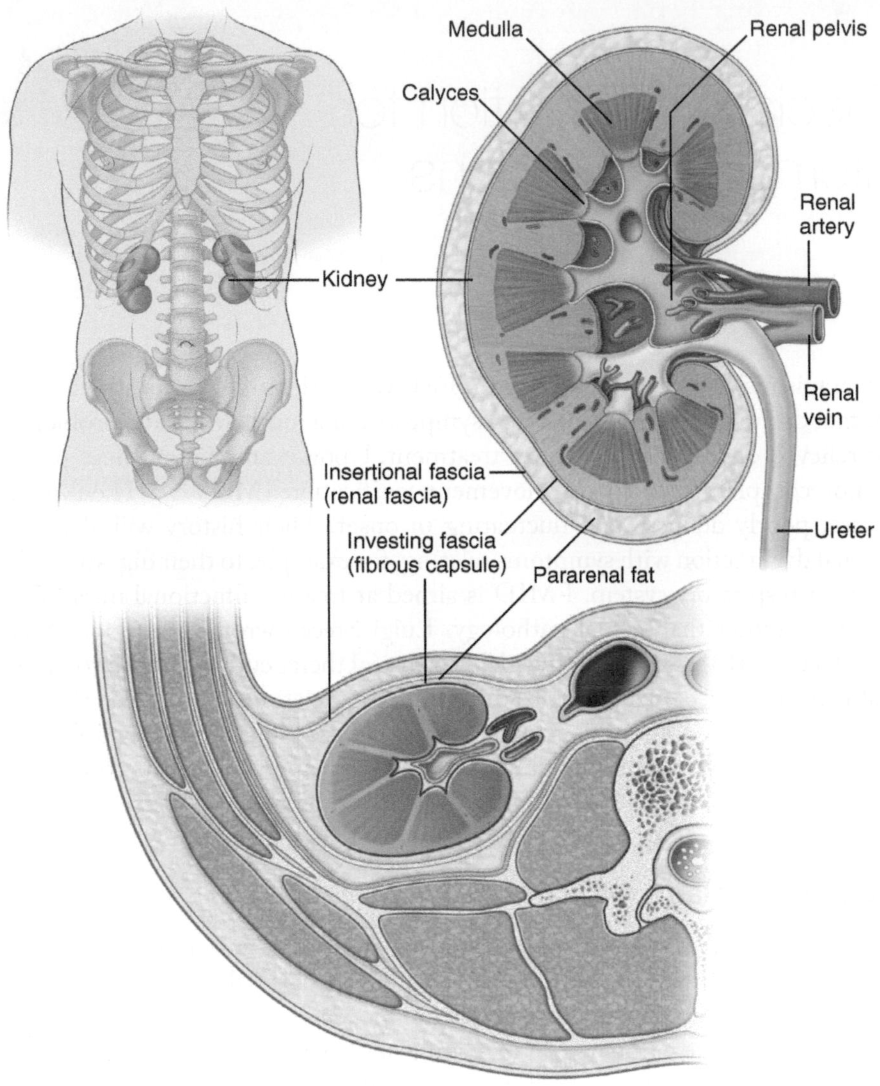

Fig. 6.1 Investing and insertional fascia of the kidney.

closely adherent to the organ. In the lung, for example, an example of an investing fascia is the visceral pleura, which has close contact with parenchyma.

Organs need to move autonomously with respect to the musculoskeletal system. Insertional fasciae keep the organs in place and at the same time allow movement. Although insertional fasciae are always partially separated from organs, they make connections between organs and the fasciae of the trunk. Insertional fasciae appear as fibrous sheets rich in collagen fibres. Insertional fasciae form (ligament-like) anchors between the organs and other tissues, for example, the round ligament of the liver. Insertional fasciae divide and connect, creating a twofold role in our body. They connect the internal system to the musculoskeletal system. Insertional fasciae can be compared to the aponeurotic fascia. It is thicker and easily separated from the organ or muscle. An example of an insertional fascia of the lung is the parietal pleura, which is free to move and has connecting links to the endothoracic fascia.

Insertional fasciae connect organs in both transverse and longitudinal directions. Longitudinal connections that attach organs are called apparatus. An apparatus is made up of synergic organs connected by the internal fasciae to form sequences. An example of an apparatus is the respiratory system's fasciae of the larynx and trachea that are in continuity with the parietal pleura. They coordinate respiratory function like phonation. Transverse connections unite different apparatus together. An example of transverse connection would be the lesser omentum, which originates from the lesser curvature of the stomach and reaches the liver, gallbladder, and pancreas. Also, the vena cava and aorta are connected to the lesser omentum (Stecco and Stecco, 2014).

The abdominal wall works as a cover for the organs and ensures their vital space. When we are moving and activating our muscles a space must be maintained for the organs. Altered tension via the myofascial system can generate compression and change the pressure within an organ's space. Because of this, FM practitioners focus their treatment on the trunk area to create and restore the space organs require. FMID is not focused directly on internal organs but toward the muscular fascia that relates to the internal fascia. The myofascial continuity of the muscular fasciae together with the internal fasciae explains why it is possible to work with fascial densifications distant from a disorder.

Tensile Structure and Catenary

The abdominal cavity of the trunk is covered by a tensile structure, which is similar to a lightweight fabric membrane that is resistant and yet modifiable. This abdominal membrane is composed of and held by supporting tensors, which are formed by collagen fibres of fascia and muscles. These supporting tensors are divided into a longitudinal (AN-ME), lateral (AN-LA), and oblique direction (IR) extending in the trunk through the tensile thoracic, lumbar, and pelvic segments (Fig. 6.2). These three supporting tensors of the tensile structures of the trunk create what are called catenaries. They form the three planes of tension that should be flexible with its two extremities anchored in fixed points. The trunk tensors (TH, LU, and PV) are anchored to what are called pivots. Pivots are distal tensor bone insertion points in the deep fascia of the upper and lower limbs. It is necessary that there is a balance between the distal tensors and the trunk tensors so that the tensile structure of the trunk remains neutral and therefore does not adversely influence the mobility of the visceral organs.

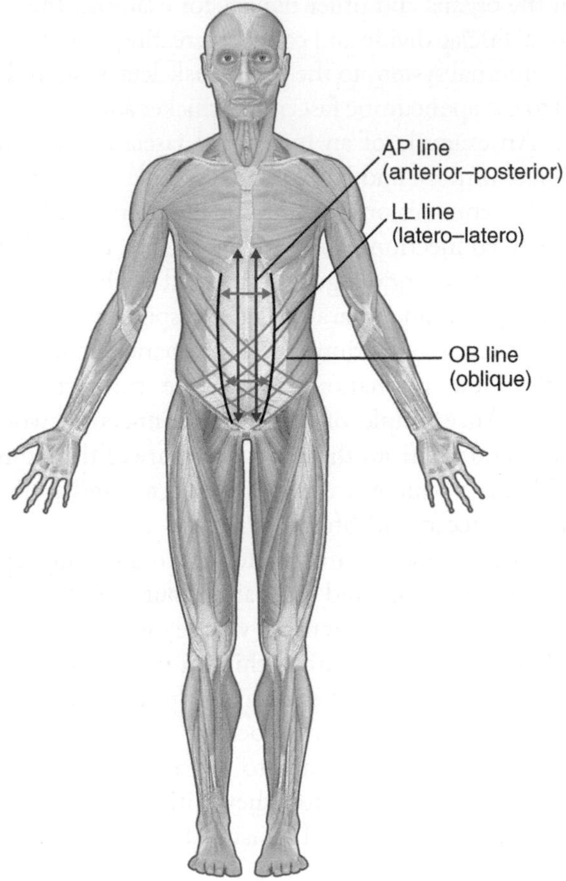

Fig. 6.2 Tensile structure formed by antero–posterior, latero–latero and oblique lines.

Basal tone and myofascial continuity create the stability and mobility of the body. Imbalance and stiffening of the tensors indicate poor adaptability of the abdominal tensors and therefore possible dysfunction of the insertional and investing fasciae. Alteration can be identified by palpation of the densification of the centres of fusion (CFs) and centres of coordination (CCs). The approach in FMID differs from the musculoskeletal FM approach in that the intent is to balance a tensile structure, including the posterior back and extremity tensors, to maintain a normal catenary. In some cases a distal tensor can compensate for tension coming from the trunk and the pain or dysfunction can be felt in the hands or feet. Our first case example, postoperative internal dysfunctions, clearly depicts this pattern. To learn more about internal dysfunction, immerse yourself in Luigi Stecco's book, *Fascial Manipulation for Internal Dysfunctions*.

Case Examples of Fascial Manipulation for Internal Dysfunctions

A few cases are introduced to help understand the concept behind FMID. We have the tools that can help more complex disorders to be understood and relieved. Many symptoms occur because of disease and some are entwined for other reasons like inactivity, dysfunctional movement patterns, or discordance between organs. Internal dysfunction after operations, premenstrual syndrome (PMS), and Ehlers–Danlos syndrome (EDS) are discussed as case examples. Many disorders can be alleviated, such as stomach problems, irritable bowel syndrome, dysmenorrhea, oedema, asthma, or reflux (Fig. 6.3).

INTERNAL DYSFUNCTION AFTER AN OPERATION

Patients can undergo appendectomy or caesarean section, hernia, intestine, uterus, and bladder operations, among others. Quite often people are not aware that there may be postsurgical implications. Some of these might show up after several years and the presence of symptoms may appear gradually. As with all patients, taking a complete history is necessary and the therapist should be able to follow the logical path of symptoms and hopefully decide on an original cause.

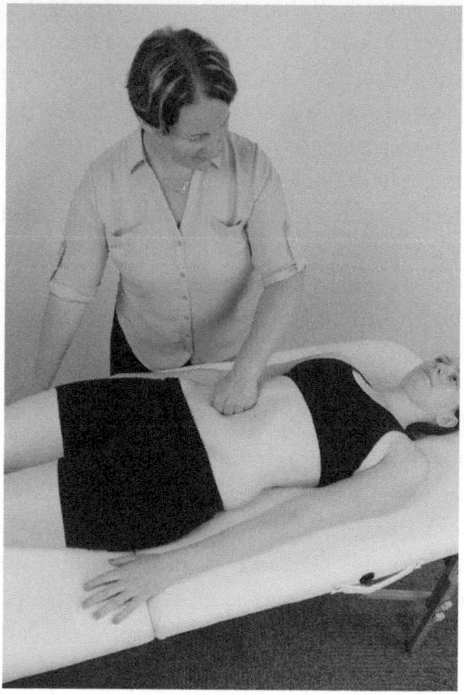

Fig. 6.3 FM treatment focused on the abdominal area.

Jane had her uterus removed 6 years ago, and her recovery was very slow. It took almost 4 months for her to get back to her work. She is 47 years old and has been suffering with low back pain and severe aching of both hips and shins. These symptoms started 4 years ago. She also complained of pain on the right side of her foot and leg during the last year. Her doctor injected cortisone to the ankle but it was not helpful. Jane is a nurse and she has been quite inactive the last few years because of her pain. She would like to walk her dogs more and start yoga or a similar hobby if her pain could be controlled. She has been on sick leave for 3 months and changes were made in her job to support her and make work a little easier. Low back and hip pain is constant and she wakes up in the middle of the night with calf cramps.

She has been taking pain medication without relief. Treatment by other therapists for her back pain has resulted only in temporary relief. Exercises have made her worse. At present she feels rigid, causing her to move in a slow manner. At the first FM treatment session we concentrated on balancing her pelvis and lower limb areas. Movement verification showed a normal range of motion for both hip and lumbar areas, but pain was present in every direction at end range. In her case, the most compromised diagonal was the antemedial, and points correlating to internal dysfunctions were also found to be painful and densified. Treatment was performed in the abdominal and pelvic areas to balance the antemedio catenary of the trunk. Balancing was created at the ankle area (segment of talus, TA). Jane felt very relaxed and tired after the treatment. She reported that after the first treatment she cried a lot and was able to sleep without cramps.

The second FMID treatment was scheduled the following week. At that time she stated that the pain has increased toward her right foot. Her abdominal area was more sensitive now. She has had pinching feelings every now and then and her groin area is bilaterally sore. She has not taken any medication. Her movements are smoother with diminished pain in her low back. Results after the first treatment session were promising and the second treatment was focused on balancing the most altered line of tension, in her case, the oblique catenary. Jane feels that FM gave her long-lasting results, although there is still a lot more to balance. Increasing her ability to maintain an active life will take time, and treatment was scheduled to support her efforts to increase workload and daily activity. After the fourth treatment Jane felt more confident and aware of her own body. She is more capable of identifying the situations that might require more energy than she is capable of.

Anatomic continuity of the fasciae of the abdominal wall, pelvic floor, and lumbar region supports the idea that symptoms in the pelvic area can travel around the body and also affect the lower limbs. When balancing tension of the pelvic floor we enhance the normal functioning of the pelvic organs, muscles, and fascial layers. Fascial dysfunction like restriction and densification can create both an internal and external imbalance. It is necessary to create a perfect equilibrium of forces to establish normal coordination, contraction, activation, and timing. Jane's prolonged pain, surgery, and scars were responsible for the increased stiffness of the fasciae around her organs and pelvic muscles. With time, tension had spread toward her right foot and in the end she had low back pain and leg pain caused by a previous operation and eventual imbalance of her myofascial system. Often the pelvic floor and limb pain are considered as two separate problems and are treated in a different manner. With the FM approach we can consider continuity between the pelvic floor and lower limb and we can hypothesize that these problems are related to each other. This approach allows us to treat several problems at the same time (Fig. 6.4).

PREMENSTRUAL SYNDROME

PMS is one of the most discomforting occurrences for a female. Women experience some of the most dramatic mental and physical changes during this time. Almost one-third of women suffer from PMS until they reach menopause when symptoms begin to fade. Physical changes can include weight gain and fatigue. Changes in fluid dynamics can lead to bloating of breasts, legs, arms, and feet. Cramps in the stomach, diarrhoea, nausea, vomiting, and headaches typically accompany this disorder. The reasons for the occurrence of PMS are not very well known. The physical reactions can be attributed to the physical changes that happen inside the body during ovulation (Imai et al., 2015; Ruy, 2015).

Symptoms that are related to PMS vary and often patients do not realize that they are connected. Often their symptoms have been treated separately with medication or sick leave. Ann, our case example, has been suffering from PMS symptoms since her first period. She gets crippling headaches, dizziness, and nausea together with accompanying mental stress. She is now 25 years old and her period started when she was 13. She works in a library and has been reading books about this matter, and finally she came up with the idea that fascial treatment may be of help. She does yoga and Pilates in her spare time, but quite often the headaches are so severe that she has to cancel her hobbies. As is often common in these cases there are no clear movement problems. She feels miserable and there is nothing that seems to ease her symptoms. Sometimes medication and exercise offer relief, but never permanently.

Based on palpatory verification (PAVE) the oblique catenary was impaired more than the others. In the pelvic area fasciae connect the rectum to the seminal vesicles and to the bladder. The broad ligament of the uterus inserts into the iliac fascia and transversalis fascia, which are in a similar continuity. Dysfunction in this area might alter pain perception and change the coactivation between different organs. An abnormal tension of the fasciae of the pelvic region can lead to incorrect activation of the system and the patient may experience stomach or pelvic problems along with pain and swelling. The autonomic nervous system is closely related, and

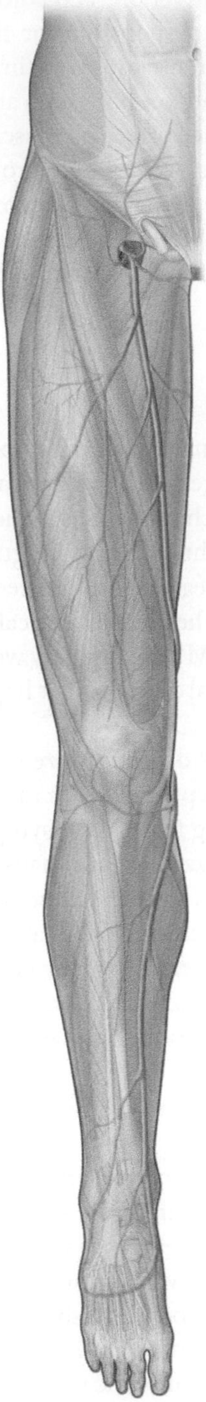

Fig. 6.4 Continuity of the fascia from pelvis to lower leg.

so anxiety and mental problems can be related, as in Ann's case. In FMID fascial disorders can affect visceral, glandular, or vascular components, and the therapist determines the combination of different systems to be treated. Ann's case required balancing the autonomic nervous system and hormonal secretion.

During treatment Ann responded with emotionally overpowering feelings and post-treatment she felt very relaxed. Treatment was started from the lumbar and pelvic area, but the head was an important factor and was added to the protocol. The neck was included because of densification between the two heads of the sternocleidomastoideus (SCM). Ann's first treatment was 1 week after menstruation, when she still complained of a headache with a visual analogy scale (VAS) of 8/10. After treatment she reported that the pain decreased to 3/10. We decided to schedule the FM treatment again 1 week after menstruation. After the third treatment session we achieved the results we were looking for. Ann did not have any dizziness or nausea after her period. Headaches were 2/10 during menstruation, and eased off in 1 week without medication. She was very happy about the outcome and when the pain was diminished, she noticed that light exercises like walking, Pilates, and yoga also relieved her symptoms during her period. Ann felt that her moods became more stable. It seems from a clinical aspect physical changes improve psychological tension. It is a common misunderstanding that menstruation is always painful and women act awkwardly during it. This is not the case. As Ann said after the treatment sessions, "seek help and trust your own body".

Pelvic pain can be associated with symptoms involving musculoskeletal, gynaecological, urological, or gastrointestinal systems without inflammation or specific pathology (Apte et al., 2012). Pelvic fasciae maintain normal tension and balance between muscles of the abdomen, back, and limbs. Dysfunction of these connections may cause alteration of fasciae in distant locations. The close connection between the autonomic nervous system and fasciae is a key element in this case. Headaches and mood changes were related to autonomic reactions and balancing the tensional patterns enhanced the synchrony of the different systems (Fig. 6.5).

EHLERS–DANLOS SYNDROME

EDS is a disorder that affects the connective tissue. Skin, fascia, bones, blood vessels, and many other organs and tissues can face failure in this disorder. Defects in connective tissues cause the signs and symptoms, which vary from mildly loose joints to life-threatening complications. A commonly used classification is known as the *Villefranche nomenclature*, and types are distinguished by signs and symptoms, underlying genetic causes, and patterns of inheritance (Knight, 2015).

Many people with EDS have soft tissue that is highly elastic and fragile. EDS patients tend to bruise easy and some types of the condition can cause abnormal scarring. People with the classic form of EDS experience wounds that split open with little bleeding and leave scars that widen over time. In some cases ruptures,

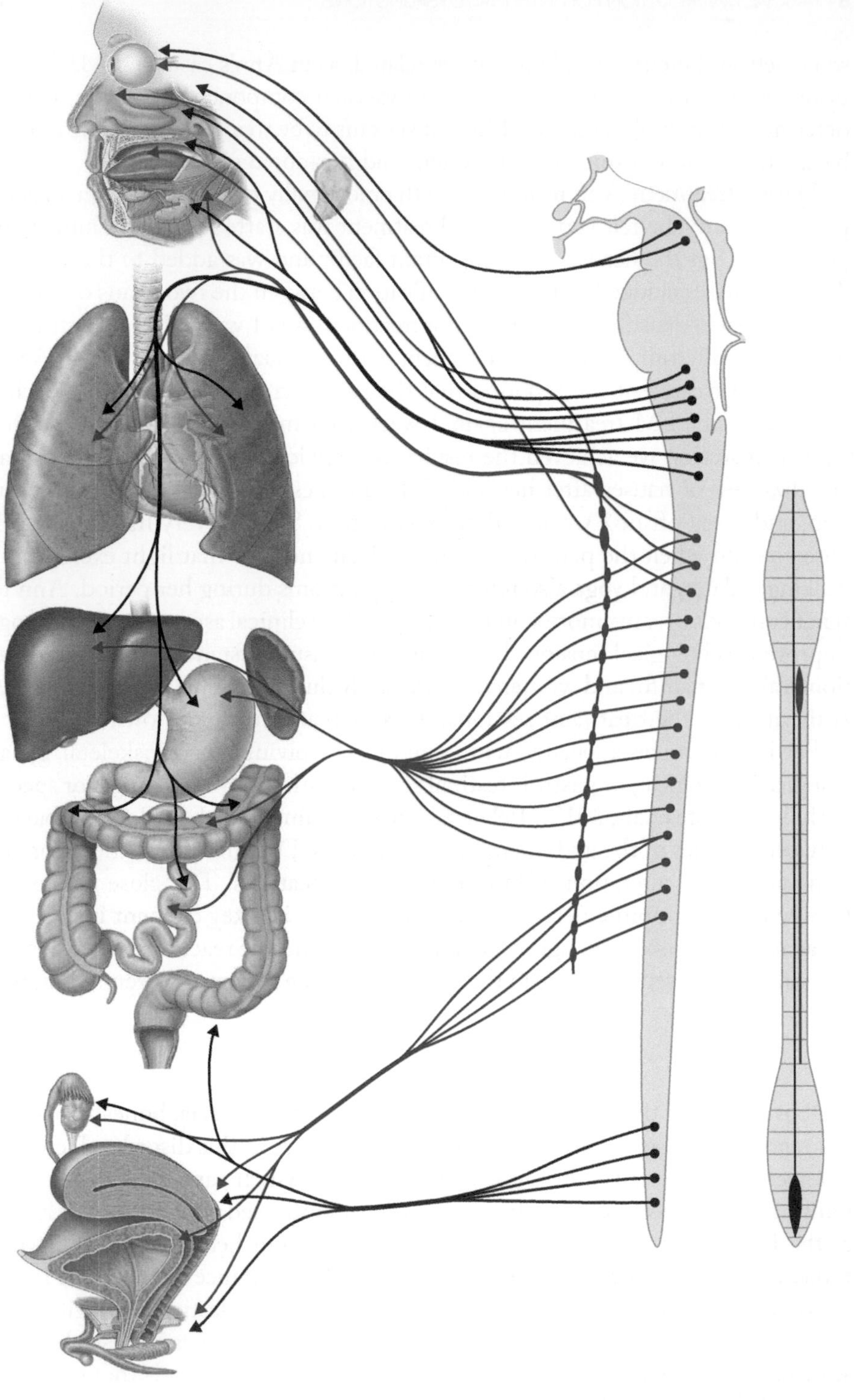

Fig. 6.5 Autonomic nervous system and its relationship to the fascial system. *(From Stecco and Stecco, 2014.)*

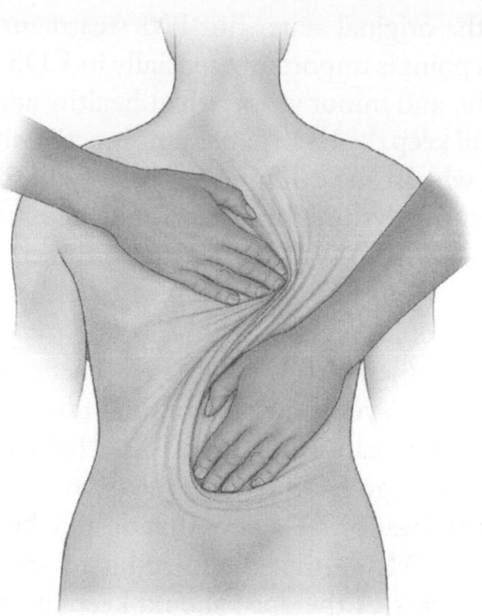

Fig. 6.6 Laxity of the skin, Ehlers–Danlos syndrome.

dislocations, hernias, organ ruptures including tearing of the intestine and rupture of the uterus, and internal bleeding are associated with the diagnosis. People with the kyphoscoliosis form of EDS experience severe, progressive curvature of the spine that can interfere with breathing. Although it is difficult to estimate the overall frequency of EDS, the combined prevalence of all types of this condition may be approximately 1 in 5000 individuals worldwide. The hypermobility and classic forms are most common. The hypermobility type may affect as many as 1 in 10,000 to 15,000 people, while the classic type probably occurs in 1 in 20,000 to 40,000 people (Castori et al., 2015; Scheper et al., 2015) (Fig. 6.6).

Sally is in her forties and has always been considered very hypermobile. She has had subluxations and dislocations in her shoulder joints and ankles. Over the years she has had luxations in her knees bilaterally and in her left elbow. Her skin is very elastic and hypotonic. She feels very tired after regular housework and works 60% of the time. She struggles after work with her normal chores at home. Pain is always present in her life and travels from one area to another. If she makes uncoordinated movements she might lose her balance or dislocate a joint. She is active in the EDS Association, and the peer support she receives seems to help her mentally.

In these cases more FM treatments over time may be required since EDS patients suffer with a variety of symptoms most of their life. FM seems to be a very beneficial treatment for them. Even though the treatment may be relaxing, patients report that their ability to move is compromised and the treatment may have been too much for their bodies. Because of hypermobile joints they do not benefit from joint mobilization or manipulation. It might help for a day or two, but their symptoms return to the original state. But FM treatment seems to support the immune system. This point is important especially in EDS patients who are more prone to infections, flu, and minor viruses than healthy adults. Reinforcement of the immune system will keep the EDS patient more active and allow them to have a more active social life, which can be diminished because of tiredness and their complex symptoms. When the dysfunctional tension is released from the fascial network, patients can coordinate movement better and feel more stable due to the proprioceptive feedback from FM. FM in these cases benefits sensory feedback and proprioceptive control in a system that is lax and hypermobile.

Sally has been seeing a therapist who has been practicing FM for several years and she has noticed that her syndrome is stable and not progressing. She has days when she is not in pain and can work and exercise lightly. She states that she is feeling better than the average EDS patient she encounters in her EDS support group. This gives her motivation to believe that despite her diagnosis she can live an almost normal life. FM is utilized according to movement and palpatory verification as in other cases. A therapist should keep in mind that these patients should not be not overtreated. Less is more. While this syndrome is incurable, using FM procedures in a modified way can ease symptoms and help patients to live better in their daily life.

FMID provides a total body effect on a fascial connecting system that influences a variety of symptoms at the same time, from muscles to organs, including the visceral (gastrointestinal/respiratory), glandular (endocrine/haemopoietic), and vascular systems. It is important to educate our patients by communicating this type of information so they will understand why they are improving without medication.

Reference

Apte, G., Nelson, P., Brismée, J.M., Dedrick, G., et al., 2012. Chronic female pelvic pain—Part 1: Clinical pathoanatomy and examination of the pelvic region. Pain Pract. 12 (2), 88–110. http://dx.doi.org/10.1111/ j.1533-2500.2011.00465.x.

Castori, M., Morlino, S., Ghibellini, G., Celletti, C., Camerota, F., Grammatico, P., 2015. Connective tissue, Ehlers-Danlos syndrome(s), and head and cervical pain. Am. J. Med. Genet. C. Semin. Med. Genet. 169C (1), 84–96. http://dx.doi.org/10.1002/ajmg.c.31426. Epub 2015 Feb 5.

Knight, I., Hakim, A., 2015. A Guide to Living With Ehlers-Danlos Syndrome (Hypermobility Type), 2nd ed. Singing Dragon.

Imai, A., Ichigo, S., Matsunami, K., Takagi, H., 2015. Premenstrual syndrome: management and pathophysiology. Clin. Exp. Obstet. Gynecol. 42 (2), 123–128.

Ruy, A., Kim, T.H., 2015. Premenstrual syndrome: A mini review. Maturitas. 82 (4), 436–440. http://dx.doi.org/10.1016/j.maturitas.2015.08.010. Epub 2015 Aug 28.

Scheper, M.C., de Vries, J.E., Verbunt, J., Engelbert, R.H., 2015. Chronic pain in hypermobility syndrome and Ehlers-Danlos syndrome (hypermobility type): it is a challenge. J. Pain. Res. 20 (8), 591–601. http://dx.doi.org/10.2147/JPR.S64251. eCollection 2015.

Stecco, L., Stecco, C., 2014. Fascial Manipulation for Internal Dysfunction. Piccin, Padua, Italy.

CHAPTER 7

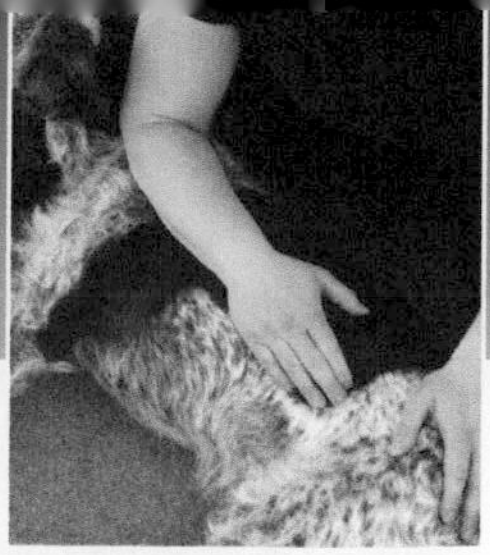

Veterinary Fascial Manipulation

Fascial manipulation (FM) also includes veterinary fascial manipulation (VFM). With few exceptions, both types of FM follow a similar protocol. Anatomic differences are unique for every species; therefore sequences, diagonals, and spirals are based on the particular species, its fascial network, and movement patterns. At present, the fascial networks of dogs and horses have been mapped by dissection and the results of this work are taught in VFM level 1 and at workshops. In order to be proficient in VFM a strong anatomic education along with knowledge of dealing with animals is necessary. Many countries have animal physiotherapists, massage therapists, chiropractors, and osteopaths who specialize in VFM. In most countries veterinarians are designated as the professionals who treat the animal kingdom (Fig. 7.1).

Indications for VFM are pain, lameness, movement dysfunction, stiffness, or coordination problems. Overall, VFM is indicated for musculoskeletal disorders. Precautions are needed when an animal has behavioural problems and, while it might be indicated to use VFM, it may also be necessary to consult with a veterinarian. In complicated situations, after traumas, operations, or injuries, cooperation with a veterinarian is mandatory. Contraindications to VFM are fever, acute infections, inflammations, and skin lesions. Animals that have successfully been treated with VFM range from domesticated dogs and cats to top-level competition horses. Most often these problems are not related to age, sex, or breed.

As in FM, VFM protocol begins with a case history. It is usually focused with the person who spends the most time with the animal. But the interpretation of the animal history may present problems. For example, domestic animals like cats and dogs often spend their whole life with the same people, while horses can have a blurred history. They often travel from one country to another and track of their history might be lost. Owners, trainers, and vets are very important partners when dealing with animals and their history. The FM assessment chart remains a useful tool when gathering information about animals. As in humans, the chart is used to record history, movement and palpatory verification, and treatment with the reassessment.

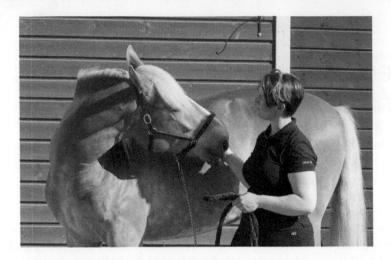

Fig. 7.1 Veterinary fascial manipulation protocol includes case history, movement and palpatory verifications before treatment. Movement verification can be performed by using treats like here in the picture with Finnhorse mare. *(Courtesy of Niina Virtanen.)*

Observation is the key element of the VFM assessment, because an animal sign language can give clues regarding pain, compensation, and origin of the dysfunction. In VFM the feeling hands are even more important than with humans, and a careful gradual examination is essential throughout the whole VFM protocol. Movement verification (MOVE) is often performed first using passive movement. VFM therapists must feel the quality and quantity of movement and compare symmetry between sides. Responses of the animal should be noted carefully. Active movements are often functionally coupled and with animals they should be observed during movement in which they encounter problems. For example, a jumping horse may refuse to jump, a dressage horse may have trouble with flying changes, or agility dogs might persistently jump in a crooked manner. If the owner or trainer is able to point out when the problem is visible, the therapist might try to provoke the symptoms. Active movements can be tested at times with treats, especially with dogs and horses. Treatment is advised to be performed first with minimal tension. Beginning with superficial palpation the therapist and animal can both tune into a similar frequency and after a connection is achieved the therapist can work more thoroughly with the animal. Deep fascial manipulation is manifested with compression and friction mainly using the fingers as a treatment tool. The animal fascial system is very sensitive and often the treatment point rapidly releases. Even with horses, only minimal force is necessary when manipulating the fascia.

The following examples highlight some of the many conditions that VFM can encounter. Just as in humans, different animal species can suffer with overuse, misuse, disuse, and trauma. VFM often solves musculoskeletal problems in one to three treatments. Many animals are masters of disguise, because in nature it would be dangerous to show weakness. The most important thing is that animals are intuitively balanced and express a natural homeostasis that allows self-healing. Treatment after surgeries is recommended with the cooperation of the veterinarian (Fig. 7.2). After VFM treatment, in general, the animal should have 1 to 2 days rest. Normal activities are possible, but heavy training should be performed 2 days after VFM treatment at the earliest. After operation the recovery time is due to the normal healing process of the body and training should begin progressively.

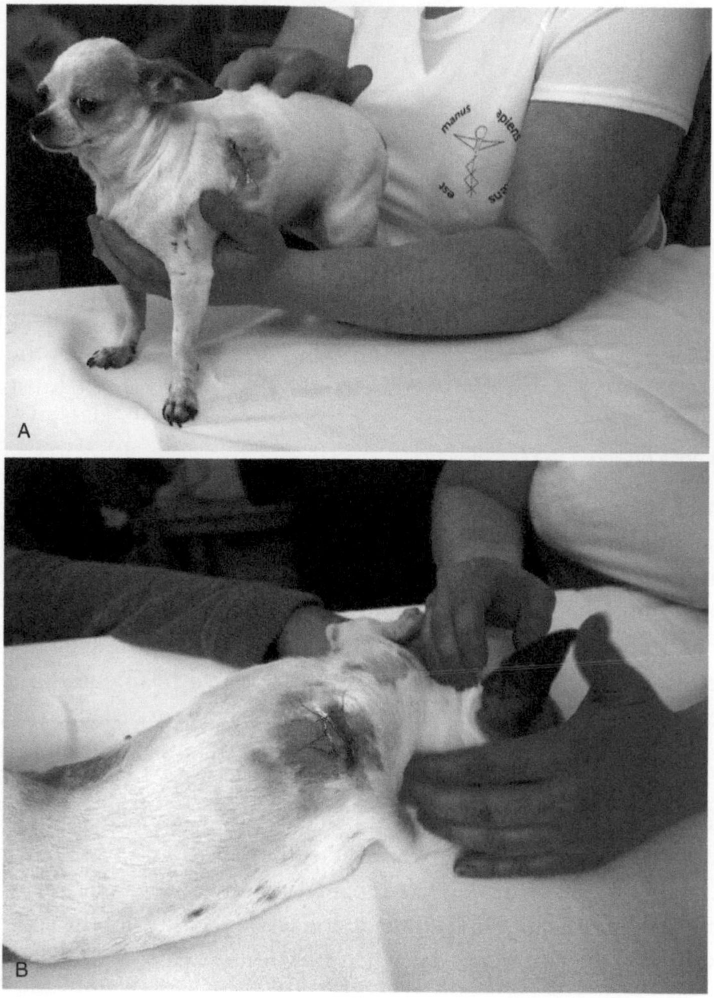

Fig. 7.2 VFM treatment after an operation includes palpation of the segments near the operation area. (A) Superficial palpation should be performed first with the fingers around the segment. Palpation of the deep fascia should be introduced gradually. (B) VFM treatment is performed side-lying in this case.

Cats

Cats are elastic movers and can compensate for minor problems that may be difficult to notice. Therapists using VFM should be aware of cat behavioural patterns. Adequate communication with the owner is essential before starting the treatment. Because of their small size, it is sometimes hard to verify the correct plane to treat cats. Only fingertips should be used in these cases.

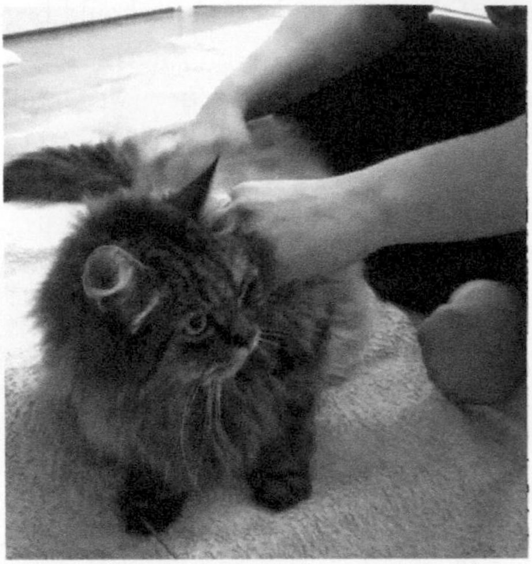

Fig. 7.3 Mimosa having a VFM treatment.

Mimosa, 8 years old, had her left hind leg crippled after she was hit by a car 2 years ago. She survived, but after the accident she ran on three legs with her left hind leg raised. Mimosa was checked by the vet, and her X-rays were negative regarding fracture or dislocation. She has been managing with the crippled leg, but 2 months ago the owner noticed that she had difficulty jumping to her favourite shelf. This was the main functional problem reported by the owner along with lameness. She has been with this owner all her life and he stated that Mimosa never experienced any previous trauma. Mimosa was behaving very nicely during the treatment and the problematic plane was verified to be horizontal. Hock area (fascia of the peroneal muscles ER-TA lt), hip (fascia of the vastus medialis muscle IR-CX lt and fascia of gluteal area ER-CX lt), and pelvis (fascia over the iliac spine ER-PV bi) were treated. After the VFM treatment the owner reported that Mimosa was able to jump up and walk on all four legs. Cats are intriguing animals, and while they are not the easiest to treat, they are willing to tolerate treatment when they sense that it is needed (Fig. 7.3).

Dogs

The breed of a dog predisposes it to different problems due to alignments and conformations. Breeding has led to breathing or moving problems in some breeds. People are also working with dogs in different fields. They can assist in the military or police services, which will require good endurance and physics. Also agility, sled, and racing dogs face the demands of force generation, endurance, and proprioceptive tasks. VFM therapists can be useful in many ways when dealing with working and sport dogs or dogs who are their owner's best friend (Fig. 7.4).

Dogs are often more straightforward to treat as they are usually pretty obedient and willing to be with humans. Our case example is a 6-year-old Leonberger called Nancy who gave birth 6 months ago. Soon after, the owner noticed that her right hind leg was always laterally rotated. Nancy is a show dog, so posing in the right position is important. She has no traumas in her history and has been with the same owner her whole life. She has been pregnant three times. Movement verification was done by observing walking and trot and then by passively checking the range of movement of the lumbar, hip, and knee area. According to movement verification the horizontal plane seemed to be the most impaired. After palpatory verification (PAVE) the treatment was planned to restore the balance of the AN-LA spiral. The alteration was continued from the right hind leg towards the trunk to the left front leg. Treatment started from anterior and lateral side of the hock area (AN-LA-TA rt) continuing towards the medial and posterior side of the knee (RE-ME-GE rt) and anterior and lateral part of the hip (AN-LA-CX rt). From this point tension changed to the left side and the point over the erector spinae

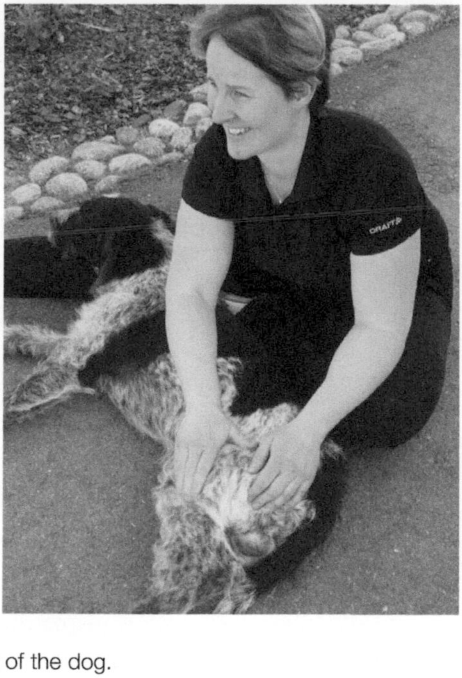

Fig. 7.4 VFM treatment of the dog.

fascia was treated (RE-ME-TH lt). The last two points were treated from the left front leg. Points RE-ME-SC and AN-LA-HU are located in the scapular fascial area). After VFM, Nancy was walking and trotting straight lines and the case seemed to have been solved in one treatment session. The owner was advised to call if the problem recurred.

Horses

Sensitiveness of horses is dependant on the breed. Warm-blooded horses are very sensitive and their nervous systems seem to be very responsive. They are fast and often used as a race horses and endurance horses. Cold-blooded horses are more often used as carriage horses and in tasks requiring endurance and increased power. Requirements for dressage, jumping, endurance, event, or Western horses vary according to tasks they need to perform. VFM therapists must develop a basic knowledge of the reactions and features of the variety of breeds. Learning as much as possible about a horse will allow you to better interpret both its movement and response to palpation. All of this information will allow the formation of an accurate hypothesis and a better understanding of the horse's reaction to treatment (Fig. 7.5).

Our example is Nicolas, a 10-year-old thoroughbred gelding used as a riding school horse. He has been moving in a crooked manner during riding lessons for the past 2 months. His right front leg has been shorter on striding, especially on the left rein. The problem started after a snow storm and the owner thinks that he might have slipped in the paddock. The history of this horse is not known, but

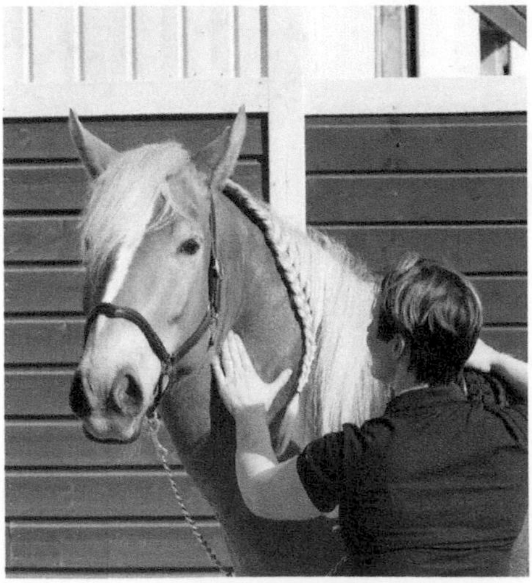

Fig. 7.5 VFM treatment of the horse. *(Courtesy of Niina Virtanen.)*

TABLE 7.1 ■ **Nicolas' Assessment Chart**

	Segment	Location	Side	History	Rec/ Const	Pain Modality
Si Pa	LU/PV	LA	rt	Slipping, 2 m	Const	Walking crooked, pelvis shifted to the right.
Conc Pa	SC-CA	AN/RE	rt	Slipping, 2 m	Const	Shorter stride in trot
Prev Pa	TA	RE	rt	Trauma, scar		Do not know the time frame

Si Pa - site of pain; Conc Pa - concomittant pain; Prev Pa - previous pain; LU/PV - lumbar and pelvic area; SC-CA - from scapula to forearm area; TA - shin; LA - located to the lateral side; AN/RE - located in anteriorly and posteriorly; RE - located posteriorly; m - month; const - constant.

there are some signs of an old injury in the right hock since a scar behind the hock indicates some trauma in the past.

Observation of gait was done first. It showed that Nicolas was shifting his pelvis to the right when he was walking. During walking his front legs seemed to move normally, but in the trot his right front leg took a shorter step. Passive movement verification of the right hind leg, bilateral lumbar area, and right shoulder were tested. Examination revealed a reduced range of left lateral lumbar movement and decreased abduction of the right shoulder. The right hind leg did not reveal any movement deficiencies. There was also a rotated pelvis present. Movement and palpatory verification incriminated the frontal plane. Palpatory verification was done to the pelvic, lumbar, thoracic, and humerus areas (PV, TH, LU, HU). Lateromotion (frontal plane) was the most densified sequence, and repeated palpation indicated that the points of the latissimus dorsi muscle bilaterally (LA-TH bi) were the most densified and painful areas (see Table 7.1).

Treatment began on the superficial gluteal muscles (LA-PV bi) and continued to the right lateral shoulder (LA-HU rt) and elbow area (LA-CU rt). After balancing these points by treating the tensor muscle of the antebrachial fascia, above the olecranon and triceps medial head and anconeus muscles (ME-CU rt). At first the point near the latissimus dorsi was so sensitive that Nicolas would not allow even minimal pressure. Often in FM, when a particular point is very densified and painful, in this case (LA-TH bi), treatment of points proximal and distal to the most tender point helps to release the tension in the sequence. This reduces the pain at the most tender area allowing treatment. Post-VFM treatment revealed that the trunk and pelvis were aligned and balanced. The quality of strides in trot seemed to be equal. Passive movement of right shoulder abduction was in normal range. The owners were told to rest Nicolas for 2 days from the riding school and then attempt normal riding activities.

CHAPTER 8

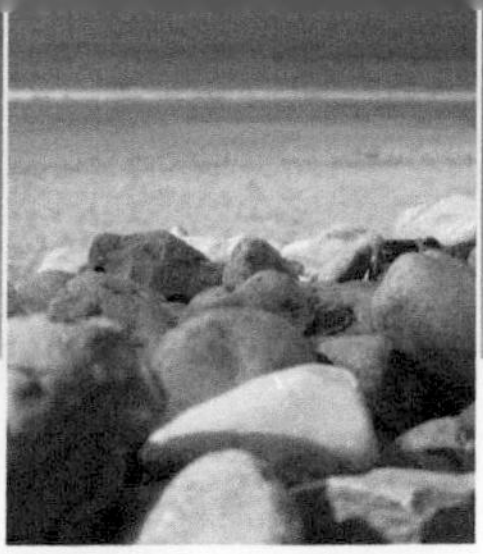

Conclusion

As A.T. Still wrote in 1899, "We begin with anatomy, we end with anatomy, and knowledge of anatomy is all you want." Without anatomy we lose our presence. We can express our feelings and emotions through our anatomy. Damasio (2010), from the world of neuroscience, asserts that our brains project our emotions and feelings by way of our body.

The idea of tensional areas in the body is ancient. Hippocrates (500 BC) taught how to perform cross-friction massage and use hands as a therapeutic tool. For ages, people have attempted to heal and enhance patient performance by the use of all types of hands-on methods (Graham, 1884). Acupuncture points from China and the heritage from the Imperium of Rome have been influential. Leonardo da Vinci (six studies of the bones and muscles of the arm in 1508–1510) was studying anatomy detail by detail. His anatomic drawings were extremely precise. Andreas Vesalius (1514–1564, the father of anatomy – *de humani corporis fabrica*) and Hieronymus Fabricius (1537–1619, the father of embryology) were teaching in Padua, Italy. Students learned anatomy in the anatomic theatre, one of the first in the world. The wings of history are still beating there today. Recent breakthroughs in the science of fascia are considered revolutionary in the world of anatomy and physiology. Its importance has been greatly underestimated over the last decades (Fig. 8.1).

Clearly, our ubiquitous fascia is a major player in our bodily actions. Luigi Stecco has helped us to understand the myofascial kinetic chain throughout our body and the importance of maintaining a normal basal fascial tone. He has been an eager gatherer of information, developing a biomechanical model of the fascial system that can be used to evaluate and treat the fascial system. Fascial manipulation (FM) has been under development since the 1980s and it is still growing. New insights, refinements, and theories continue to influence the FM model. Based on dissection and anatomic studies, the Stecco family continues to improve and amplify FM. Scientific fascial research is expanding every year, with already over 1000 published peer-reviewed articles. Ongoing anatomic, histologic, and clinical studies will continue to expand our understanding of this multidimensional tissue.

Healthcare practitioners are important from the patient perspective. Disorders, dysfunction, pain, stiffness, or loss of function can be improved by manifesting FM. This method provides an answer to the question: "Why do I have pain?" It validates a global way of thinking and combines fascial anatomic knowledge with bodily function. FM has proven to be a brilliant contribution to practitioners and their patients (Fig. 8.2).

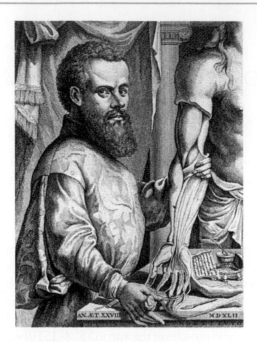

Fig. 8.1 Andreas Vesalius, father of anatomy.

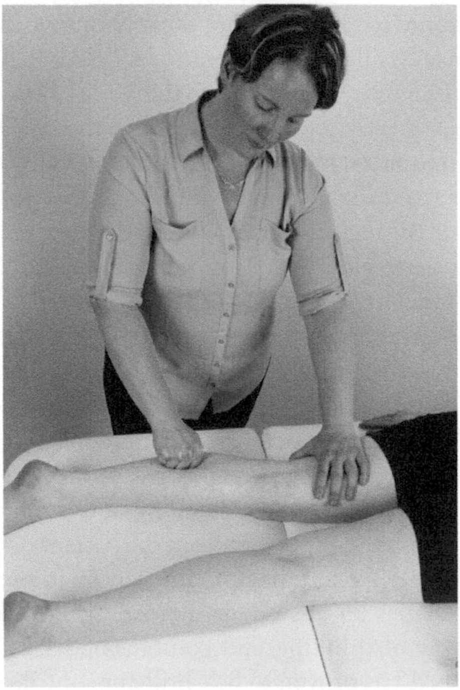

Fig. 8.2 *Manus sapiens potens est*. Treating hands can be powerful tools.

References

Damasio, A., 2010. Self Comes to Mind: Constructing the Conscious Brain. Deckle Edge.

Graham, D., 1884. Practical Treatise on Massage: Its History, Mode of Application, and Effects, Indications and Contra-Indications; With Results in Over Fourteen Hundred Cases. Reprint: Forgotten Books, 2013.

INDEX

Note: Page numbers followed by *f* indicate figures, *t* indicate tables, and *b* indicate boxes.

Printed and bound by CPI Group (UK) Ltd, Croydon, CR0 4YY
03/10/2024
01040470-0005